Additional Praise for *A Guide to Body Wisdom*

"[Brode] brilliantly distills all of her breadth and depth of experience in this surprisingly practical book. Readers will be richly rewarded with accessible counsel on how to tap into the wisdom of the body to enhance health and well-being."

—Michael Seabaugh, PhD, clinical psychologist

"In Ann Todhunter Brode's new book *A Guide to Body Wisdom*, there's room for curiosity and satisfaction, space to expand and contract as one sees fit. The book invites us to be present in each moment as we notice with awareness our bodily sensations and our thoughts and then consciously decide how we want to think, feel, and react."

—Nancy Eichhorn, PhD, founding editor-in-chief of *Somatic Psychotherapy Today*

"A vital resource for people who hope to live a balanced life and to feel fully alive."

—Richard Louv, bestselling author of *Last Child in the Woods*

"A priceless guide to living a healthier life. [It] can help you change unhealthy behavior in an empowering and educated way. A must-read for anyone who wants a healthier body, mind, and life."

—Aleya Dao, author of *Seven Cups of Consciousness*

"Beyond [Brode's] amazing work as a practitioner, she also possesses a breadth and depth of knowledge about the body/mind connection of great use to anyone seeking a better life for themselves and others."

—Aaron Kipnis, PhD, Professor Emeritus, Pacifica Graduate Institute, clinical psychologist, and author of *The Midas Complex*

"In *A Guide to Body Wisdom*, author, healer, and therapist Ann Brode takes a refreshing and inspired approach to your health and well-being…She offers valuable insights and a wide variety of easy-to-understand methods to connect with your body's wisdom. This is a wonderful, down-to-earth, practical road map filled with many helpful ideas and step-by-step techniques to help you love and reconnect with your body so you can live a happy and healthy life."

—Pamala Oslie, author of *Life Colors* and *Infinite You*

"It is a joy to see a seasoned practitioner in our field craft such a careful book to create the possibility for many more people to experience the intricate and profound body practices that we have been so blessed to find in the nooks and crannies of our dissociated world, with the amazing benefits derived from them. It has enough materials to engage one for a long time."

—Don Hanlon Johnson, PhD, founder of the Somatics Graduate Program at California Institute of Integral Studies and author of *Diverse Bodies, Diverse Practices*

"Brode's perspective is long overdue, offering a holistic, balanced view of what it means to be human."

—Larry Dossey, MD, author of *One Mind*

"Ann Brode based on her 30 years of practice as an extraordinary healer, has written a masterpiece of insights, meditations and exercises that illuminate the wisdom of the body. She shows us how to deepen our practice of body awareness and how to align our mind and spirit … this book will become a classic in the literature of our conscious evolution toward a more enlightened, body-centered awareness and compassion."

—Dr. Craig F. Schindler, JD, PhD, former professor at UCSC, president of Project Victory, and founder of the Wisdom Intensives

"[This is] must reading for every person who has ever felt sick and tired and doesn't know how to reboot and refuel. Rooted in compassion, rich with solid self-care, and written by someone who has heard every body's story, *A Guide to Body Wisdom* is a true treasure of life-changing information that will assist anyone in healing their body and their life."

—John La Puma, MD, *New York Times* bestselling author of *ChefMD's Big Book of Culinary Medicine* and *The RealAge Diet*

Disclaimer

The material in this book is not intended as a substitute for trained medical or psychological advice. Readers are advised to consult their personal health care professionals regarding treatment. The publisher and the author assume no liability for any injuries caused to the reader that may result from the reader's use of the content contained herein and recommend common sense when contemplating the practices described in the work.

This book is not intended to provide medical advice or to take the place of medical advice and treatment from your personal physician. Readers are advised to consult their doctors or other qualified health care professionals regarding the treatment of any medical problems. Neither the publisher nor the author take any responsibility for any possible consequences from any treatment, action, or application of medicine, supplement, herb, or preparation to any person reading or following the information in this book.

For Dennie.

a guide to
Body Wisdom

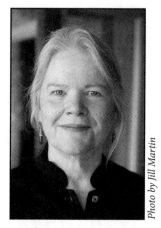
Photo by Jill Martin

About the Author

Ann Todhunter Brode (Santa Barbara, CA) has focused on the relationship of body, mind, and spirit as it shapes the physical experience for more than forty years. As a teacher, therapist, healer, and writer, Ann is a respected leader in the bodywork community. She has written for *Health Source Magazine, Santa Barbara Independent, Huffington Post,* and *Somatic Psychotherapy Today Journal.* Visit her online at www.AnnTodhunterBrode.com.

To Write to the Author

If you wish to contact the author or would like more information about this book, please write to the author in care of Llewellyn Worldwide, Ltd. and we will forward your request. The authors and publisher appreciate hearing from you and learning of your enjoyment of this book and how it has helped you. Llewellyn Worldwide, Ltd. cannot guarantee that every letter written to the author can be answered, but all will be forwarded. Please write to:

Ann Todhunter Brode
℅ Llewellyn Worldwide
2143 Wooddale Drive
Woodbury, MN 55125-2989

Please enclose a self-addressed stamped envelope for reply,
or $1.00 to cover costs. If outside the USA, enclose
an international postal reply coupon.

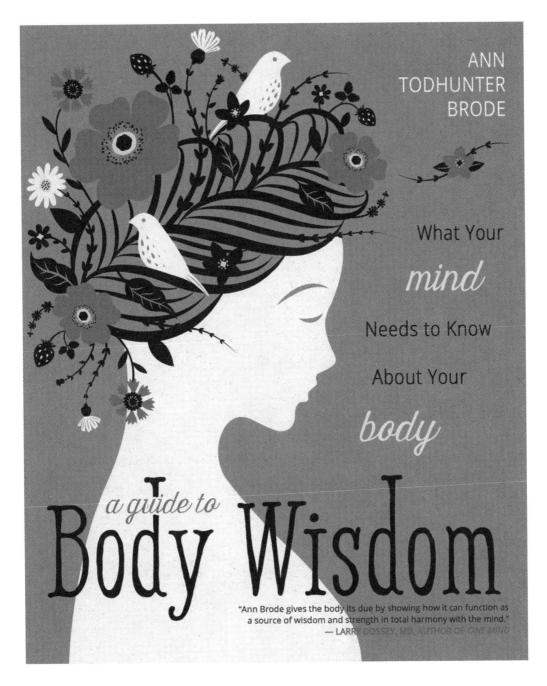

ANN
TODHUNTER
BRODE

What Your
mind
Needs to Know
About Your
body

a guide to
Body Wisdom

"Ann Brode gives the body its due by showing how it can function as
a source of wisdom and strength in total harmony with the mind."
— LARRY DOSSEY, MD, AUTHOR OF *ONE MIND*

Llewellyn Publications
Woodbury, Minnesota

FIRST EDITION
First Printing, 2018

Book design by Bob Gaul
Cover illustration by Yulia Vysotskaya/Deborah Wolfe Ltd.
Cover design by Shira Atakpu
Editing by Laura Kurtz

Llewellyn Publications is a registered trademark of Llewellyn Worldwide Ltd.

Library of Congress Cataloging-in-Publication Data
Names: Todhunter Brode, Ann, author.
Title: A guide to body wisdom: what your mind needs to know about your body/
   Ann Todhunter Brode.
Description: First edition. | Woodbury, Minnesota: Llewellyn Publications,
   [2018] | Includes bibliographical references and index.
Identifiers: LCCN 2018007455 (print) | LCCN 2018014904 (ebook) | ISBN
   9780738757216 (ebook) | ISBN 9780738756950 (alk. paper)
Subjects: LCSH: Mind and body therapies.
Classification: LCC RC489.M53 (ebook) | LCC RC489.M53 T63 2018 (print) | DDC
   616.89/1—dc23
LC record available at https://lccn.loc.gov/2018007455

Llewellyn Publications
A Division of Llewellyn Worldwide Ltd.
2143 Wooddale Drive
Woodbury, MN 55125-2989
www.llewellyn.com

Printed in the United States of America

Contents

Exercise List

FOUR: Stress and Relaxation

FIVE: Healing

EIGHT: Body and Spirit

Acknowledgments

All of the mind-body pioneers mentored my early years as a motor perceptual therapist. For pointing the way, I am especially indebted to the brilliance of Carl Rogers, Morris Berman, Moishé Feldenkrais, Ida Rolf, Ron Kurtz, Mary Whitehouse, and Charlotte Selver. It was my good fortune early on to study extensively with one of the best—Judith Aston. Judith helped my healing gift become a practical reality and has remained an inspiring and long-time friend.

Over the years, I've had the pleasure of working with amazing clients who've trusted me to guide them on a journey of learning, healing, and transformation. Without their insights and discoveries, this book would have no substance. As often happens in the course of a therapeutic relationship, my clients became my teachers and healers.

Although writing is a singular and sometimes lonely pursuit, no one writes a book alone. The inspiration for this book came from a place beyond that could be called the Divine Muse. The process, itself, was a steady learning curve assisted by the input and patience of my techie family, savvy writer friends, and various professionals along the way. For their patience and humor, I thank Carrie and Thomas Paine. For responding readily to artistic requests, I thank Emma and Chris James. For their reliable counsel and emotional support, I thank Ben Eichenberg, Tracy Cabanis, and Gail Steinbeck. For her insights, tips, and companionship on the journey, I thank Susie Meserve.

In addition, I want to acknowledge my copy editor, Kimberley Litherland, for her impressive precision. And, I'm eternally grateful to my writing coach and content editor, Ilene Segalove, who saw the potential and helped me sculpt the raw material into a finished product. Through each draft, Ilene patiently prodded me onward to find practical, accessible, and result-oriented ways to bring the wisdom to you. As my dear early readers, Michael Seabaugh and Ann Wisehart, can attest, this book has come a long way.

Stepping into the world of publishing, Gareth Esersky at the Carol Mann Literary Agency, offered enthusiasm, encouragement and hand-holding. The professional excellence of Angela Wix, Kat Sanborn, Laura Kurtz, and the team at Llewellyn made it easy to feel confident and participate in bringing this book to the world.

Along the way, I was touched by the generosity and enthusiasm of Larry Dossey, MD, and Guy Claxton, PhD, who valued this book as a worthy contribution to the body-mind-spirit lexicon.

My list would be incomplete without a big thank you to all my dear ones who've had to hear about my book for years… and especially my husband, artist Benjamin Brode, who cooked the dinners and kept things going when I was tethered to the computer every weekend, all weekend.

Foreword

Ann Todhunter Brode started her training with me in 1973. Over the years, I have witnessed her learning, teaching, pondering, and generous sharing with her clients and students. As a gifted teacher and writer, Ann has developed brilliant ways to help people listen to, understand, respect, and work with their body's innate wisdom. *A Guide to Body Wisdom* is an impressive self-help book designed to offer her effective techniques and vast experience to many others.

Even if you have a shelf full of self-improvement books, you'll want to read this one. This is why: Over the past twenty years, health and wellness books have changed the way we *think* about our bodies. These books often overlook the possibility that the body might possess an intelligence of its own—a unique wisdom that could get on board and help us be smarter in every aspect of our lives. *A Guide to Body Wisdom* gives you all the guidance and information you need to change this mindset and build a new, healthy relationship with your body.

Yes, it can be challenging to change thoughts and behaviors shaped over a lifetime, but the importance of this book couldn't be more profound. When stress, multitasking, and virtual reality seem to have sidelined the body, putting it front and center becomes a viable way to return to balance and sensibility. Let this book introduce you to a body-mind relationship that just feels natural. Such an alliance is truly one of your most valuable assets.

Ann Todhunter Brode has written a book that fleshes out the missing half of the mind-body equation. The depth of her understanding, vision, experience, and communication skill make her an excellent facilitator for transformational growth and healing.

It is with great pleasure that I invite you to start or continue your journey on page one.

Judith Aston-Linderoth
Creator and Director of Aston Kinetics

Introduction

Just think—your body and its gene pool connect you to a lineage that goes way back to the first humans who walked on earth. Take a moment to imagine how essential it was for your ancestors to read signs of danger, find sources of food, identify healing plants, and build adequate shelter. Such skills and knowledge not only assured their comfort, they determined their survival. In the most basic way, your body has always held the bottom line and the key to a successful, healthy, and fulfilled life.

Even though so much has changed over the last hundreds of thousands of years, your biological imperatives remain unchanged. If anything, success and survival have gotten a lot more complex. For instance, a couple of centuries ago, most people were aligned with nature. They had few choices and were physically active all day long. They ate locally, labored steadily, went to bed with the sun, and woke up with the birds. Nowadays, things are different. There's a lot of sitting, a lot of thinking, a lot of worrying, and a diminished connection with the native intelligence of the body. Perhaps when people stepped away from the forests and fields, their body wisdom went to sleep.

Once you reawaken your body's innate wisdom, you'll be impressed by what it has to offer. Learning how to pay attention and listen is the first step in making good lifestyle decisions and designing personalized care programs. The Body Wisdom IQ Test will help you evaluate where you are right now and inspire you to make some changes. Some of the changes are basic things like nutritious food, good exercise, and replenishing rest. Next, you may be asked to move on to supportive environments, stimulating challenge, intimate relationships, and spiritual connection. *A Guide to Body Wisdom* is designed to lead you back to your essential body and give you the tools to take care of this valuable asset. Taking care of the basics now will set you up to survive and thrive in the future.

Getting the most out of life might be simpler than you think. Contrary to popular belief, living a full life doesn't mean mega drama and burning the candle at both ends. Listening to your body will help you dismantle one of the biggest threats to health, happiness, and longevity—stress. Not only are your body basics similar to those of your ancestors, so is your flight-or-fight wiring. Did you know that your physiology has a similar response to both a lurking saber-toothed tiger *and* a near miss on the freeway? Even an important job interview can make your cortisol levels spike, muscles clench, and heart pound. Such intensity is very useful if you need to get away or defend yourself every once in a while. But when a jar drops in the supermarket or you're playing a first-person shooter video game, your adrenaline can begin pumping as if that tiger was truly nearby! In the fast-paced, high-stimuli, 24/7 world of today your body may be constantly triggered and hard-pressed to find any peaceful interludes. This is neither healthy nor enjoyable. *A Guide to Body Wisdom* will help you recognize what's going on, cultivate a baseline for relaxation, and develop body-oriented strategies for diverting the intensity of stressful times.

Whether it's a seasonal flu, a broken bone, or a devastating disease, your body is there to help whenever you find yourself suffering. Getting in touch is invaluable anytime you want to improve your health or need to heal. Not only can your smart body be a guide and comfort when you're sick, injured, or off your game, it's also the place to start when you need to heal old wounds and establish new routines. This book will help you listen to your body when you ask the questions: Am I as happy and healthy as I'd like to be? Am I suffering the symptoms of long-term neglect and chronic overload? Is a recent injury reminding me that it's time for a break? Or, how can I be more proactive with a chronic, complicated health issue? To return to true health, resiliency, and balance takes more than pharmaceuticals and protocols. In order to be healthy and stay healthy, you need to listen to your body. And when your body is aligned with mind and spirit, you have a dynamic equation for self-healing.

Even if your body feels healthy right now, your disquieted emotional life might be tripping you up or holding you back. Ongoing despair and discord take a lot of energy and distance you from life. To be alive is to have feelings, and these feelings live in your body. Joy and delight are on a spectrum of emotions that include anger, sadness, and fear. Your body can help you identify, understand, and express these emotions. From your body's point of view, moving emotion is just another natural physical process like relaxing tension, releasing toxins, or breaking a sweat. When you embody your emotions, they're no longer mysterious; they're simply part of being human. *A Guide to Body Wisdom* will teach you how to be more emotionally aware *and* emotionally intelligent. This is the key to living inside your experience and participating in the poetry of life.

This book will help you follow your body's wisdom to find authenticity, confidence, and success. This is how it happens: as you become more rooted in your body, you feel more confident; feeling more confident, you begin to speak from your inner-truth and listen with your inner-knowing. What you say has an assured authority, and what you hear is reinforced (or not) by what you feel. Your interactions begin to have a satisfying intimacy and reliable accuracy. This book includes many time-tested, body-oriented suggestions to empower your intentions, improve your communication, and deepen your intuition.

Your body is your natural home. From basic needs to individual quirks, when you know yourself, you have the inside scoop on health, happiness, and living fully. How reassuring to have such a sounding board and trustworthy source so close at hand! Even when you ask esoteric questions or seek philosophical answers, your body has something to offer. As long as you're alive, spirit is incarnate. Knowing your body intimately and feeling its spaciousness are important bridges to your spirit sense. Crossing that bridge is the finishing flourish that truly makes living artful and graceful. This will be reflected everywhere in everything you do. Let this book take you on a progressive journey to discover, cultivate, and enjoy your body wisdom. It will change you and how you live in the world.

How to Use This Book

Over the past four decades, people have asked me to help them with body issues. They want to be comfortable, healthy, happy, and successful and they wonder if some bodywork might be a good place to start. *A Guide to Body Wisdom* represents the experience and learning of all the people who've come into my studio. Now, I have written it down with you in mind, as if you just walked in my door.

As with any new client, we'll begin at the confluence of interest, need, and opportunity. Something inspired you to pick up this book, so let's keep going as we invite your body to wake up and take the lead. This will be easy if you imagine that your mind is the seeker, the book is the personal trainer, and your body is the master guide. Together, we'll systematically dismantle unproductive behaviors, attitudes, and assumptions, and find ways to assemble the building blocks for healthy living. Your learning will be tailored to your personal interest, reinforced through a multitude of examples and exercises, and paced at your own tempo. In this way, your insights can lead to new ways of seeing and being. As the gridlocked tension and habitual patterns let go, stored emotions move on and new truths appear on the horizon. *A Guide to Body Wisdom* is an invaluable resource to help you systematically release restrictions, integrate new information, and find comfort in the present moment.

Although each person's experience will be different, there are some basic truths and reliable pathways to unlock your body-voice, access your body-intelligence, and cultivate your body-wisdom. It begins and ends with how you live in your body. Chapter by chapter, as you unravel the history and personal mythology stored in your sentient body, you'll have a clearer picture of where you stand and where you're going. Along the way, you'll discover ways to cultivate and enjoy your body's great potential.

Overview

To get a scope of the journey ahead, let's take an overview of where you're going. *A Guide to Body Wisdom* is designed as both a teaching and therapeutic experience with a multitude of ways to help you begin to live consciously in your body. Just like someone coming to my studio for help, it works best to approach the book with an open mind and proceed at your own pace. Throughout the book, I typically use first person pronouns, because I am writing this for you, the reader/seeker. I have included intriguing scientific, psychological, and personal stories to help your mind understand what we're up to. Throughout, you'll be encouraged to participate in the various experiential exercises to clarify concepts, illustrate new ideas, and solidify your learning. Remember, it takes practice to change old habits, embrace new attitudes, and establish new routines. Once you awaken your sentient, intelligent body, you can access its profound wisdom anytime you need it.

Each chapter is a sequential increment in a therapeutic progression. For this reason, even if you hunt and peck at the beginning, you'll want to eventually read the book cover to cover. Skipping to the troubleshooting index at the back of the book or skimming over topics that don't seem pertinent to your life right now is one way to personalize your experience, but don't miss out on the various exercises and activities! The on-the-spot check-ins (Try This) are a fun and informative way to experience some of the concepts firsthand. The more extensive processes (Explore) are included to help you find deeper understanding and do some self-healing. As you explore, keeping a separate Body Wisdom journal will help you reflect on your discoveries and record your insights. As with all new learning, the important stuff will stick and the rest will fade away for now.

No matter what reason brings you, this book will introduce you to your most valuable asset—your wise body. In these times of extraordinary change and challenge, having some body wisdom is a good way to manage stress, stay resilient, and make accurate decisions. Reading this book will help you use all your resources, be responsive to the world around you, and remain true to yourself. How reassuring it is to be able to trust your own body as a guide and ally.

Getting Started

What if you opened this book for a reason? To find the answer to this question, simply ask your body: "What do you need?" Then tune in, create a bit of open space, and the answer will pop into your head. Perhaps you:

- Want to change some habits, do some healing, be more resilient
- Need to learn how to love yourself, let go of the past, be intimate
- Would like to let go of self-criticism and negative thinking
- Want to reap the fruits of your labor and show up for love and joy

Listen to your body and honor what you hear. *A Guide to Body Wisdom* will help you help yourself.

To begin, you'll want to read the chapter entitled Waking Up to change your mind and get aligned with your intelligent body. Then, you may want to address some specific concerns. For instance, if you're dealing with chronic pain, check out the chapter on healing; if you're dealing with hypertension or sleep problems, check out the chapter on stress and relaxation. Be sure to review the troubleshooting index at the back of the book where I've highlighted common issues and concerns that bring people to my therapy practice. Each situation has a precise recipe of readings and exercises to personalize your learning. Like many people, however, you may have been intrigued by the title of this book and want to know about more body wisdom. In that case, simply start at the beginning, read chapter to chapter, and enjoy your sequential journey to transformation and healing.

Truthfully, this book is so chock-full of gems and tidbits that you could open it at random in the morning, read a paragraph, and have something to ponder all day long. Once you get started, you'll learn a lot of fascinating things and begin to see your body from a different viewpoint. From this new perspective, you can see what's missing, what's off-track, and what needs to heal. *A Guide to Body Wisdom* gives you the information, tools, and perspective to help you find the health, fulfillment, and body wisdom you've been looking for. This is the beginning of a fun, enlightening, and rewarding adventure.

And, Afterward

Reading this book will help you find yourself anew and embrace your wise body at last. Long after you've finished reading, it'll be one of your most valuable reference books. Whenever you find yourself in a time of question, challenge, or change, pick it up to refresh your knowledge, learn new things, and do some personal body-oriented therapy. No matter how unhooked or unhinged you feel, you can trust this book to lead you back to your steady source—your body wisdom.

One
Waking Up

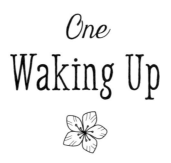

While you use your smart mind every day, you hardly use your smart body at all. Even if you're moving around, physically fit and functioning, there's more you need to know about living in your body. Did you know that your body holds an innate intelligence and ancient wisdom that is wholly separate from your mind? This part of you has been there all along. Yet if your thinking mind dominates the scene, it probably feels as if your body is dumb or numb. To access your full potential, you need to wake up and really feel your body. You can then begin to use your smart body's vast resources for awareness, vitality, healing, balancing, communicating, intimacy, intuition, and quality of life.

For most of human existence, life needed to be oriented around physical experience in order to survive. But as less time was spent in nature (hunting, gathering, and surviving) and more time was spent pondering the nature of things, the primacy of the body began to diminish. In the seventeenth century, Descartes argued convincingly for the separation of psyche (mind) and soma (body), and since then, the body has been relegated to something mechanical and devoid of intelligence, personality, or spirit. As scientific studies focused on the body machine (digesting, working, performing, reproducing), the connection to the sensible body (experiencing, reflecting, connecting, knowing) went to sleep. Now, in the twenty-first century, we need to take another look at the body and wake up in order to survive.

Using the latest technologies and cutting-edge physics, scientists are unraveling the mysteries of the body and finding a new application for the old adage that the whole is greater than the sum of its parts. Take a look at a bio-imaging scan or biochemical map and you'll see an intricate link between psyche and soma, mind and body. In addition to a magnificent machine, the evidence seems to imply that your body is also smart. It's time to change your mind and cultivate some body wisdom. To do this, you don't have to go into a lab for proof or understand a complex equation. All you have to do is shift your perspective a bit and pay attention to the obvious.

Start at the Beginning
How Do You Relate to Your Body?

Take a moment right now and see where you stand with *your* body. Do you feel intimate and comfortable or distant, disappointed, and awkward when you focus on your physicality? Do you trust your body as an ally and reliable partner, or do you need to direct and manage it all of the time? Are you as kind and loving to your body as you are to a dear friend? Do you speak about your body in ways that reflect respect and understanding? What you say and think about your body could be perpetuating old belief systems. To see where you really stand, ask yourself one more question: "Do I trust my body to guide my decisions?" Your answers tell you a lot about the status quo. Follow your relationship with your body over the next few days and you might be surprised. When you say *me*, do you mean your body, as well as your intellect, personality, and feelings? When you talk about your body are you possessive (my arm, my movement) or objective (the jaw, the illness)? Do you feel insecure about your health and need reassurance from professionals for the slightest disturbance or discomfort? Do you see your body as something that needs to be managed, corrected, and improved?

The way you think and talk aren't random. Listen to yourself. Your words can tell you a lot about your intimacy, connection, and identity with your body. Here are some reasons why it's important to wake up and pay attention to the words you use:

- Your body is listening to everything you say and think.

- When you dismiss your body, you diminish the potential for health and happiness.

- When you boss or bully your body and deem health and fitness as chores, you're negating a willing and eager partnership.

- When you criticize your body for genetic or circumstantial imperfections, you're implying that it's the enemy and not trustworthy.

- When your words aren't inclusive and respectful, your body wants to check out.

- When your smart body is out of the picture, you aren't cultivating your most valuable resource—body wisdom.

In order to change the program, you need to change your tone. Stop dissing your body— end the dismissing, disrespecting, and disregarding. Start "inning"—including, incorporating, and investigating. This is a big paradigm shift. It means your body is *you*. It means relating to yourself and the world from the *inside*. This is a brand new approach and something you'll need to practice.

If suggesting there's more to being awake than getting out of bed, going, and doing seems like a riddle from Wonderland, you're not alone. To your mind, the idea may seem like a fuzzy dream or mere semantics. Don't be discouraged. *Waking up* is a simple segue from here to there. *Waking up* is seeing the world from a different angle. *Waking up* changes your perception and presents new insights, new creativity, new solutions, and renewed enthusiasm. *Waking up* is a new way of living in your body. Slowly but surely as you wake up, your mind will start to understand your body and be delighted with its new partner. Slowly but surely as you wake up, your words will begin to reflect a new respect. Slowly but surely, your feelings will register compassion and love for your body. Your body is the untapped resource that offers you the input and expertise that will guarantee true health, happiness, and fulfillment.

What's Happening Now?

Pause for a moment to drop in and see how your body feels; close your eyes and look inside; tune in to your sense of space and sensation. This is your kinesthetic sense and we'll be talking a lot about it in this book. Feel what's happening inside and ask yourself the following:

- Am I comfortable?

- Is some part of my body tightened up, squeezed off, or tucked under?

- Is my belly moving with each breath? Does this feel easy and rhythmic?

- Are my hands gently holding or tightly clutching the book?

- Is my primary focus in my head?

- Is there more awareness in my upper body than my lower body?

- Do I feel my pelvis on the chair, my feet on the floor?

As you do this body survey, notice what your mind was up to. In addition to recording the physical sensations and pondering the questions, was it carrying on a conversation of its own? Was it surprised? Did you learn something new? Did your mind seem to doubt, judge, or dismiss this exercise? Maybe your mind needs something to do.

Give Your Mind Something to Do

Your mind likes to be busy. Let it follow its natural inclination to observe and evaluate while you explore the talents and intelligence of your body. As you read, pondering new concepts and participating in intriguing exercises, invite your "curious observer" mind to follow along. Let it be enticed by the fascinating facts, anecdotal stories, personal discoveries, and novel approaches. Let it evaluate what works for you or what doesn't work for you. Some topics covered in this book may resonate, others may amuse, and still others may be completely off base for now. Your mind and your experience will help you sort out what's relevant and useful. This is what makes A *Guide to Body Wisdom* so very personal.

🌸 *Explore: Body-Home Tour*

Take a few minutes to be in body-space and take your curious mind on a tour of the premises. Imagine you're visiting different rooms of a house as you go from your head to your neck to your upper chest, et cetera. As you pause along the way and take stock, make a note of varying qualities—awareness, comfort, familiarity—and answer the following questions:

- Are some places so remote that it is hard to gain entry?
- Do some places feel more welcoming than others?
- Are some places bright, shiny, warm, cozy, dusty, or cobwebby?
- Are some places holding emotions or memories you'd forgotten?
- Do some places have something they need to say or want you to hear?
- Does the whole place seem numb or empty or overly crowded?

There's a lot of rich information here. What did you discover about yourself? In a profound way, your body holds your story. Even if it feels numb or blank or it couldn't sustain your attention for more than ten seconds, your Body-Home Tour is telling you something. Record your experience in your Body Wisdom journal. If you want, you can draw an outline of your body and color different areas to represent your findings; even your drawing has something to tell you. Jot down some descriptive words to note how you felt as you toured your interior spaces. Be sure to include anything that surprised you and everything your body had to say. Taking this tour gives you an idea of the work to be done and a reference point for comparison later on.

Touring your body home is a spot check you can do anytime. It's like checking in with your authentic inner self. You might be surprised by the depth and complexity of your body's truth. For instance, the experience could have been the first time you explored the territory and had a delightful adventure … or you might have felt awkward, silly, or self-conscious. Along the way, you may have found whole areas that were relatively silent, isolated, and dormant—as if in a deep sleep. You could have stumbled upon some old memories and long-forgotten associations. You could have uncovered places that felt wary and reticent; maybe others were tight and nervous. You might have sensed some stubbornness or defensiveness here or there. All of it has a story. Many body therapists believe that the body acts as a storage chamber for your personal history. No matter what, how you live in your body home has something to tell you, and it's a very personal message.

Everyday Awareness

Your body has been with you every single day of your life. It's easy to take something so familiar for granted. In order to see and feel clearly, it may be time to take a fresh look. All you need is sensory awareness. Your eyes are already trained to glance at every mirror you cross, so take a look. *See* what your body is telling the rest of the world about your comfort, effort, or self-esteem. What do you hear? *Listen* to the sound of your feet as you walk, the sound of your hands on the keyboard, the sound of your voice in conversation. Open your ears and listen to the sound of your patience, emotional state, or confidence. Tune in to space and place with your kinesthetic sense. *Feel* the emotional resonance and intuitive message. Let your curious mind utilize this sensory input to evaluate the inner-outer dynamic.

Your everyday awareness lets you know if you're in sync or out of touch. It helps you match your body effort to the task at hand. For instance, sometimes it makes sense for your muscles to be pumped for a difficult task; other times it makes sense for your muscles to be more relaxed and pliable for an easy load. Paying attention will help you adjust when it's leisure time and your muscles are still geared up for heavy lifting. Being aware of your body also helps you match your expression and responses to the emotional tenor of what's happening. Tune in to your sensory body for good guidance and intuition. For instance, if your stomach is full of butterflies or your jaw is clamped down, your body knows what's going on. If there's danger afoot or love in the air, your body knows what's going on. Waking up is paying attention.

Being Present

A good time to tune in and be present is at the beginning of the day, the beginning of sleep, or the beginning of anything. No matter what you're doing, pay attention to your body and you become more aware. Take a minute or two to see, feel, and be present in your body when you shift from one activity or place to another. Beginning a task or conversation with body consciousness makes it a fresh and full experience. So, let's start with the beginning of your day.

- What is your morning routine?

- Do you get nudged from sleep by the sound of an alarm clock and move into your day creaky and groggy?

- Do you gradually get it going as you shuffle through washing, dressing, eating, and morning news?

- Do you steel yourself and crash out of bed hurrying around like a mad person on steroids to meet the deadlines and match the intensities of the day ahead?

If you change your routine at the very start of each day, it changes the trajectory for the entire day. Perhaps tomorrow instead of being on autopilot, you could give yourself time to let your body wake up before you get up. This simple change could make a huge difference in how your day proceeds. No matter what's on the schedule, wouldn't it be more agreeable to start your day in your body with ease and lightness? Give it a try. Remember, how and where you begin a journey determines where and how it'll end.

Try This: Wake Up, Loosen Up

Instead of popping out of bed in your usual manner, take a few minutes (like three) to wake up to the day and wake up in your body. At the very moment your mind begins to stir, send it directly to the world of your senses. What do you hear, smell, see, and feel? Your senses are the bridge between your body and the external/internal worlds. Now bring your focus to your inner space and begin to move each part of your body gently through its natural range of motion. Start with your fingers and toes and let the movement spread to include your ankles and knees, wrists and elbows. Let each part move in its own way (including your eyes and jaw) until you've loosened up your whole body. Now you're ready to get up. You're beginning your day, bringing your awake-and-aware body with you.

Another natural time to tune in is when you're going to sleep. This is the beginning of your rest cycle. Here, rather than enlivening each part of your body, you'll want to quiet down and relax. Just remember, when you get into bed, get into your body! Try this out tonight. It's a tried and true way to let go of the day and set the course for a good night's sleep. Let your mind focus on your body as you check through to make sure it's comfortable. Then, scan around searching for pockets of busyness, intensity, and tension. Jiggle or breathe into these pockets and let them release. Your breathing can help you let go of density and fill up with lightness. With each exhale let go of the remnants of your day (physical tension, emotional issues, ideas, problems, and projects). Don't worry—if you need it, you can pick it all up again tomorrow. Feel the comfort and cozy support of your bed with each inhale. (Note: if your bed isn't comfortable, *do* something about it!) Feel your muscles melt and your bones float along on the gentle motion of your breath. Paying attention to the beginning of sleep is a good way to enter a restful, nourishing sleep.

You can tune in and check in with your body at the beginning of anything. As you shift gears in your busy schedule, go from one task to the other, or transit from the parking lot to the office building, bring your conscious body along with you. It's a new beginning whenever you take on a new task, start an interview or assignment, skirt a roadblock, need to change course, or tackle an emotional issue. Instead of plowing through these times on autopilot, use your everyday awareness and bring your body along. It just might have something helpful to offer.

Checking In

As you go through your day, check in now and then with your body. For the time being, in order to wake up, you'll need to practice some body awareness. Pay attention as you note how you think, feel, and live in your body. Listen to your body and invite it to be a part of whatever you're doing, because this is about developing a new skill. Like most people, your body is probably on automatic pilot most of the time. Your mind sets a course for action and your body simply does it. Following are some in-between times to wake up and practice body awareness:

- Anytime you're waiting in traffic, in line, or at the doctor's office

- When you're listening to a friend, the news, music, or children playing

- When you're watching a sunset, the TV, a movie, or birds in flight

- When you're walking from car to office, in the park with your dog, or at the beach

✿ *Try This: Random Body Checks*

You may be surprised to discover what's going on in your body while your mind is off thinking and strategizing. To increase awareness of your body, where it is, what it does, and how it feels, take some time over the next few days to do the following:

- Check out what your feet or hands are doing when you're waiting or idle.

- Monitor tension in your stomach or jaw during an emotional conversation.

- Observe what your tongue is doing while you read this book.

- Measure the tension in your neck and shoulders while driving.

- Feel the map of tension when you're faced with a deadline.

If your body isn't engaged in physical labor, why is it poised for action? If you want to communicate confidence, why is it so nervous? If you intend to be effective, why is it so checked out?

Your Conscious Body

When you begin to be more aware of your conscious body, everything you do will be affected. Naturally, taking care of yourself will be easier and have a higher priority. You'll know how to get healthy and what to do when you're injured or sick. Work, play, and rest will be more satisfying. Your own wise body will be a resource when you encounter challenging times, and since your body moves slower than your mind, life will slow down. You'll actually have time to be in the moment and enjoy it.

Waking up and developing body consciousness may also uncover some old wounds and issues. As long as you're unaware, unfinished, or uncomfortable, your unfinished business may just feel normal. But once you make the connection and feel the drag, you'll want to do some house cleaning. Pause for a moment right now and reflect back on your Body-Home Tour. Did you run into any clutter, numbness, blockage, or resistance that may have emotional roots? Your emotions aren't separated from your body. They're the expressive link between your body and mind. And, when they're repressed and buried in your body, they live on and on in your body…wreaking havoc! Ask yourself if some of your body's current issues (discomfort, tension, pain, numbness, weakness) have an emotional overlay. I often tell clients that the pain could actually be the *pain*. Paying attention to your body shows you both the work and the way to your emotional healing. It's worth the effort. Clearing out the past means you can stand on the threshold of your future.

When you *wake up* and get to know your body, you establish a good sounding board for decision-making. Your mind can make a case for just about anything, but the choices you make will either resonate with your body or not. As long as you're oblivious to the signals coming from your body, your mind (will and desires) calls all the shots. But, once you feel resonance in your body, your choices of food, exercise, scheduling, partnership, investment, aesthetics, and more will reflect your body's wisdom. Your body will either say yes or say no, it's that simple. Test this out. The next time you want to make up your mind, check in with your body. When you consider a particular option, does your body feel pulled toward or pushed away? Let your body weigh in and you'll make more successful choices and fewer mistakes.

When you *wake up* and get to know your body, your confidence and self-esteem will improve. Not only will your body help you know what you want, it will help you get it. It's easy to be sure of yourself when your feelings, words, and intentions are in sync. Communication has a reassuring authority if it's aligned with your body. For instance, if what you're saying carries the authority of your body, your words will be grounded and clear. If enthusiasm and certainty resonate with your posture, your eagerness will be convincing. If loving words come from your open chest, your sympathy and compassion will be felt. No matter what words come out of your mouth, the nonverbal message comes through loud and clear from your body. If the message doesn't match the body, it's unsettling and confusing for you and everyone else.

Once you *wake up* and live in your body, you show up for life. As the spiritual counselors and motivational speakers say, "The only moment that counts is the present moment." Your body is your ticket to be in *this* moment. This is why many approaches to higher consciousness strive to quiet the overactive mind and engage a mindfulness that is focused on sensual experience: breathing, sounds, mantras, and so on. These techniques are based on the idea that paying attention to your body and engaging in word-thoughts are mutually exclusive. Try it out.

❀ *Try This: Your Breathing Body*

Put this book down and close your eyes. Tune in to your interior space and relax a bit. Now, string together five breaths, inhale and exhale, and keep your sole attention on your body breathing. Notice when your busy-bee mind starts buzzing—did your focus drift away from your breath? If you keep your focus on your breath, your mind will be quiet, yes?

Your mind just can't be aware of sensory input and word-thoughts at the same time. Focusing on the simple sensations of breathing helps your curious mind circumvent your analytical mind. Once you start to describe the sensation or experience with words, however, your mind has taken over again! When this happens, tune back in to your aware body to get in the present moment and quiet your mind again. Being in the moment is both a gateway to serenity and an essential element for intimacy and intuition. Here, your quiet, spacious body can be a bridge from sensory to extrasensory perception.

Expanding Your Understanding

The everyday way you live in your body tells you a lot about who you are and where you've been. It tells you about your attitudes, self-talk, feelings, tensions, attractions, and shortcomings. Your body is you. Not only does it hold the shape of your past, it continues to shape the future. Your body has its own separate intelligence and you can use it to expand your understanding.

Like many people, when you tune in and connect with the gifts your body has to offer, your first response might be: *Why* has it taken me so long to find something so obvious? *Where* and when did all the shaping and shutting down take place? *How* can

I use this precious information to find out more? Answering these questions is a good way to understand why you've been asleep for so long. If you look at the long trail of human history, at the beginning you'll see many years of pure physicality with food, shelter, and survival ruling the day. When humans had these essentials managed, they began to be more mental—thinking and analyzing, inventing and devising. For much of recent history, the scope of the mind has seemed limitless, superior, and smart … while the body was viewed mostly as a liability—inferior and dumb. In recent years, science and technology have blown this way of thinking wide open with new findings about the interplay of body and mind. There are even some studies that suggest your stomach has a mind of its own. This is a good time to re-evaluate your assumptions and explore the new frontier of living in a wise body.

Where Did It Come From?

Perhaps, similar to legend of Rip Van Winkle, who took a nap and ended up sleeping for one hundred years, waking up may mean reuniting your mind and body after a long sleep. You might wonder what happened. Finding your body hobbled with tensions and burdened with outdated attitudes isn't just a historical/philosophical disconnect between mind and body. It affects the very way you live and breathe each day. There could be some very real reasons why you feel numb and on guard. It's logical to wonder where it all came from. The formation of your particular attitudes, tensions, and habits is a cultural story, but it's also a personal story. In order to catch up and cultivate your full human potential, you'll need to look at how your family, life experience, and culture have influenced how you think and live in your body. In a very real way, everything that affects you *shapes* you.

✺ Try This: The Shape of History

To see *where* your personal history lives in your body, remember something significant and emotional from your childhood. Your memory could involve a mega-theme (betrayal, abandonment, cruelty, trauma) or be simply circumstantial (minor injury, hunger, childhood loss, or illness). Remember how you felt and how your body reacted to this event or situation. Let your body take on the likely tension of this event. Is the shape of this tension familiar to you today? Is a defensive posture still armoring your shoulders and back? Are your legs still carrying the tension of wanting to flee? Is your belly still contracting with the recoil from pain? In times of tension or trauma, the body returns to its familiar response pattern over and over again. This is how your personal history has shaped your life. Another person will have a different history and a different pattern of tension. Freeing up this "shape of history" is a major theme of this book and will be covered in depth later on.

Your body's not just carrying the template of your immediate personal history—your familial history has an influence as well. Formative physical and emotional influences (nature *and* nurture) have literally shaped you over centuries. *Waking up* is not just noticing how uncomfortable or unconscious you are in your body today, it's also waking up the ghosts of the past and feeling where they live in your body. As you unravel the story behind your postures and habits, don't be surprised if you uncover some assumptions, attitudes, and beliefs that took root before you were even born. These generational holding patterns and agreements need to be deconstructed in order to liberate your ideas and expectations, as well as your muscles and bones.

✿ *Explore: History Leaves an Impression*

What are some historical elements that shaped who you are? Take some time to think about it and give yourself permission to speculate and fill in the blanks. You don't have to go all the way back to ancient history. Just imagine a generation or two. What were the formative events and emotional circumstances that touched and shaped the lives of your parents and grandparents? Remember the stories and look at old photographs. Get out your Body Wisdom journal and construct a family tree of your key predecessors. Jot down a few notes as you ask the following questions:

- What was the theme running through their story (hardship, fame, betrayal, exile)?

- How might this have shaped the way they felt about themselves, their prospects, and their future?

- Did these circumstances leave them beleaguered, arrogant, defensive, or fearful?

- How could this experience have influenced the way they walked in the world?

Now, pick an important person in this lineup and describe their particular circumstances. Imagine how the emotional impact of these circumstances might have impacted their body and self-image. This is easy if you bring your own body into the picture. Just put the story of your grandfather/father/mother on like a coat and let their history shape your jaw/shoulders/back. How does this feel, physically and emotionally? Now, make a sketch of what you felt in your journal and shade in areas where the family history carries on. Where does the shape of their history live in your body today? Maybe some of this (tension, attitude, posture, and so on) doesn't actually belong to you.

Often, familial tension patterns are both unconscious and repetitive. We learn through imitation and one generation passes it down to the next. Each family has its own variation like a fingerprint, and carries tension (emotional and physical) differently. Scanning the old photographs may have shown you yours. It is an important point of departure when you realize that the way you walk through the world took shape before you were even born. In order to stand in your full stature and walk unencumbered, you'll need to wake up and take off your ancestral suit. Here's how Joan used her family album to recover her true playful self:

> *Joan questioned why she always felt driven to succeed and at loose ends whenever she was on vacation. In her body, purposeful activity felt safe; casual fun felt awkward and scary. Exploring her family history told her the underlying story. Joan's ancestors, like many, had worked hard to make a better life and held strong philosophical beliefs about "idle hands." For her people, having fun was self-indulgent and suspect. As she scanned through the family photo album, she saw grim expressions and squared-off shoulders. Both men and women in the photos looked like they had never known a day of frivolity in their lives. They probably hadn't. This look was familiar to Joan. She saw it every morning in the mirror. In order to soften up and lighten up, Joan needed to shake history off her shoulders and release the habitual scowl from her facial muscles. Just shaking and smiling helped Joan free up her workhorse body and discover its playfulness. Her old photos had shown her where it all began so she could shake off the shape of the past.*

Of course you're not only shaped by your family's history and predisposition, you're also shaped by anything that impresses you. This could be an older sibling, teachers and coaches, celebrity and fashion, friends and lovers, and the seemingly random course of injury, success, illness, and attraction. It might be enlightening to take a look at these and add them to the underlying story you've just recorded in your Body Wisdom journal.

You are definitely on the way to waking up when you can track the shape of tension in your body to its underlying story. As you've discovered, some emotional events, family history, and influential relationships have a tendency to grab hold and live on way past their due date. Once you wake up, you can clean up and free up your body. Like sorting through the closets of your house, when you jettison what doesn't fit, you won't have to schlep old baggage from the past. You'll feel lighter and more relaxed. Without the historical overlay, you'll be able to work better, play spontaneously, and show up for life as your own unique creative person. Although old patterns might feel entrenched and hard to budge, you'll be delighted to know that your body was designed to change, grow, and heal.

Work in Progress

Cleaning up and freeing up doesn't mean we're all going to look or move alike. You'll still be yourself. You'll have your unique postural expression, individual personality, and a familiar muscular tension. You won't lose your sense of self, you'll just loosen the mold a bit.

Becoming conscious of your postural patterns and habitual attitudes does not mean trading them in for some template of mechanical correctness. It means embracing your body as a work in progress. As you wake up, you'll change but you won't lose the art of being you. You'll add the benefits of more choice and less rigidity, more ease and less "dis"-ease, more consciousness and less helplessness. Just think, if you unlock the hold of habit and history, you might find two or three (or twenty) more ways to express yourself, do your work, be creative, approach opportunity, enjoy pleasure, or find happiness.

Watching the fluid movements of a baby's body gives you an idea of how muscles and bones are innately designed to move easily from one expression to the next, gracefully and resiliently. Like a baby, you have the potential to be responsive in the present moment and open to the future. This is a good goal. As psychologists and health professionals have discovered, this kind of resiliency and spontaneity is equated with happiness and wellness. Stuck behaviors and rigid bodies correlate with emotional distress and illness.[1] For more than fifty years, mind/body healers have been touting the importance of cleaning up and freeing up, saying that disease is simply stagnation and "not being at ease."

Now that your body has your attention, it's time to pay attention. Understanding the situation in the context of the whys and wheres, you're probably eager to mitigate the past and explore how you can live fully in present time. Your body knows the way. Invite your curious mind to follow along as you take a fresh look at how you do things, and remember that you're a work in progress.

How Do You Stand?

Your posture is more than physical alignment and muscular tension. Your posture is also how your body represents you. It determines not only how you see yourself but also how the world sees you. Even though it may feel set in stone, waking up your posture invites options. After all, if your body was meant to be rigid and set in its ways, you'd have more calcified parts. Your body was designed to move fluidly, respond accurately, and access the full awareness of your senses. When old habits, emotional experiences, cognitive beliefs, and unfinished business get stored in your soft tissue, the resulting postural/muscular tension will hold you back. Waking up your posture is about having options.

You can even see the burden of unfinished business just by looking around. Check out the postures of perfect strangers on the street or in the marketplace. To be comfortable and respectful in your observations, you'll want to do a quick scan or use your peripheral vision. Could the postural expression you see be an emotional statement? Does it communicate a certain attitude? Go ahead and play junior psychologist—construct the underlying story of what you see. Imagine you're looking at actors on a stage. Can you identify the collapse of disappointment, the armor of fear, or the clench of anger? Now, take a look at a candid photo of yourself and apply the same scrutiny. Unless the source for anger, disappointment, apprehension, etc., is in the frame, the bodies you're looking at

---

1 "Stress Symptoms, Signs, and Causes," *HelpGuide.org*, accessed May 2016, www.helpguide.org/articles/stress/stress-symptoms-signs-and-causes.htm.

are carrying the past (even if it was as recent as twenty minutes ago). As you go through life, it's hard to be open to new things and be in present time when your body is at cross-purposes—living in the present yet holding onto postures from the past.

Make no mistake, your postural expression has a lot to say. Even though the communication may be nonverbal and bypass the cognitive mind, it influences what people think and feel about you. How does this happen? There's a whole lot of information that reaches the brain through instinctive and intuitive channels. As part of your survival wiring, this information tells you whether to trust or distrust, to move closer or further away, to embrace or reject, and so on. These seemingly subtle differences profoundly affect all decisions, attractions, and beliefs. The body is one huge nonverbal broadcaster. You pick up postural statements from other people and they pick them up from you. Waking up your posture is about clear communication.

✿ Try This: A Postural Tutorial

Stand up in place and feel how your feet interface with the ground. Think of your body as a multistoried structure, and maximize your base as you distribute your weight evenly through your whole foot. Now imagine that each part of your body stacks one upon the other from bottom to top, like the different floors in a building. As an architect would tell you, "You'll have the support you need with a good foundation and stability when the top is aligned with all below." Check your alignment many times during the day, even when sitting because the foundation includes your pelvis and feet. Make sure that your posture is giving you the support and stability you need. Once you veer away from this alignment, it'll be easy for gravity to pull you into an old habit (slouch, brace, curl, or tilt). Notice how you feel with aligned versus collapsed posture. What impression or nonverbal message do you think your posture habit conveys to others?

Brian. For many years, Brian's parents told him to sit and stand up straight. He thought this was simply a matter of manners, but when a personal trainer told him that his postural habits influenced his ability to perform and present well, it gave a whole different spin to the issue. He had a PhD in Earth Sciences but had never applied the "form follows function" principle to his own body. Not only did his new body awareness serve his future, but coming out of the slouch made a good impression in job interviews.

If you're tuned in to your posture, you have a choice. You can let go of the old habits and line up with your best self. You can also be a lot more comfortable as you release unnecessary tension in your scrunched shoulders, tight glutes, and pinched lips. Standing up for yourself happens automatically when you wake up your posture. *Waking up* means being on top of your game.

How Do You Move?

By now, you've lived long enough that your ways of moving are well-worn pathways. Paying attention to your body lets you evaluate the efficiency and comfort of your movement patterns. After all, how you move is where your mind and body partner up for action. Being mindful of your moving body's routes and routines will help you observe how conscious (or not) you are in the most mundane activities. To do this, you'll need to turn on your kinesthetic sense—your "body sense" that registers place and space in your body. Even with your eyes closed, this sense informs balance and movement.

Your kinesthetic sense was in place and recording information when you were in utero and at birth it was already pretty well established. Because it's always been there, this body sense can easily be overlooked. But, just as your auditory sense helps you hear things accurately, your kinesthetic sense helps you move gracefully and know where you are in space. People with good timing and coordination (athletes, dancers, actors, and physical laborers) have a highly developed kinesthetic sense. And, people who are klutzy and awkward often have a diminished kinesthetic awareness. Whether gifted kinesthetically or not, you can always improve this sense if you use it. Activities like yoga and tai chi improve function, self-image, and balance in large part because time is spent tuning in to the "body sense."

✿ *Try This: Do You Have Body Sense?*

An effective way to evaluate your body sense is to take vision out of the equation. Simply close your eyes when you brush your teeth or find a light switch in the dark. Let your body sense direct these activities rather than your sense of sight. You may be surprised by how unsure and uncoordinated you feel at first. If your body (kinesthetic) sense is seldom used, it becomes dull, movement is unconscious, and you may feel detached from your body. Over the next few days, tune in your body sense when you tie a shoelace, wipe down the kitchen counter, or touch a loved one. Like a skill that gets rusty, you may need to practice a bit.

To be aware of how you move and move with awareness keeps you focused on the task at hand, whether it's physical, mental, or spiritual. Your sensible body is the doorway to your smart body. No matter how trivial or complex the task, whenever you want to be more alert, efficient, and graceful, just tune in to your body sense. Track your movements throughout the day and make sure you invite your moving body to come along. When you towel yourself off, hand papers to a colleague, pet your dog, or get into your car, let your whole body participate. Some things to be aware of:

- When you turn to look over your shoulder, does your whole body turn or just your neck and head?

- When you wipe down the counter in the kitchen, do you use your whole body or just your arm and hand?

- When you stoop down to pick something up, do you bend your knees and hips or just from the waist?

You may think it saves energy to use fewer body parts when you move, but the opposite is actually the case. Haphazard, sloppy, or abbreviated movements indicate that your body sense is sleeping. The old adage "use it or lose it" applies to your body sense.

In order to reconnect with your moving body, experiment with some new routes and routines over the next few days. For instance, if you usually turn right when you go into a store, try going left. If you go to the fresh produce area first, try frozen foods instead. If you put your left leg in your pants before your right, do the opposite. If you always open a door with your right hand, try your left. If you walk along one street to the subway, walk along a different street. Challenge yourself to find equally good alternatives to the ways you habitually move through life. Waking up means being in life.

Changing Your Mind

In order to wake up and be a loving steward of your body, you may need to interrupt a subliminal message and change the way you think. Listening to your internal dialogue and hearing what you say to your body can reveal subconscious beliefs that keep you stuck and disconnected. In order to change the way you live in your body, you need to change how you think about your body. Your mind/body relationship is your most complex and long-standing relationship. It has been shaped, set, and reinforced by years and years of interaction. Some of the ways you relate to your body were even formed without cognitive awareness. They were simply downloaded from your family and culture. Just like postural habits, thinking habits can be limiting and destructive. One important strategy for waking up is to change your mind/body relationship. But first, you'll need to know what's up.

In order to identify what needs changing, take a few moments to ponder how you think about your body:

- Are you the coach and your body the (reluctant or star) athlete?

- Are you the parent and your body the (obedient or spoiled) child?

- Are you the boss and your body the employee, underling, or servant?

- Are you good buddies? Or, are you strangers?

- Are you reliable partners? Or, do you feel at odds with your body?

- Are you compassionate and trusting companions on life's journey?

Your body/mind relationship probably has many facets and they all stem from how you think about your body. But unless you are compassionate and trusting companions, your body often ends up being dominated and dismissed by your mind.

❀ *Try This: Listen In*

Begin to notice the words and phrases and expectations you hear when you talk about your body: appearance, talents, style, abilities, habits, appetites, and so on. Self-talk is so habitual that you probably didn't even realize how pervasive it is. For now, don't judge or try to change anything, just notice the words you use. Write them down in your Body Wisdom journal so you can reference them later. This is your very own unique collection of self-perpetuating, hypnotic messages. As you read on, you'll learn ways to rewrite the script so you can truly cultivate and access your deep body wisdom.

Words are powerful and formative. To change the way you think about your body, you'll need to change the way you talk to/about your body. It's hard for your body to be smart when your mind keeps sending the message that it's stupid, stubborn, lazy, weak, or simple. It's hard for your body to become wise if it never has a chance to show up and deliver. It's hard for your body to feel appreciated when your words negate its beauty, perspectives, and talents. The message your mind broadcasts is like a trance chant that keeps your body subdued and asleep. The internal language you use shapes and perpetuates how you feel today *and* how you'll feel in the future. Tune in and you might be surprised to hear the pervasive and unproductive "notes to self" that get transmitted daily. Waking up means taking control.

Feeling Emotions

When you wake up your sensory body, you feel your feelings more clearly. After all, emotion happens in your body: your scared belly flutters; your angry jaw clenches; your happy heart swells. Part of waking up is feeling where and how your emotions live in your body. Of course, the assignment can be challenging when emotions (even joy and excitement) feel unsettling, uncomfortable, or unacceptable. Chances are, since you were very young, you've asked your body to do the impossible and hide your feelings. You've buried, blocked, hidden, sidelined, squeezed off, and tried to forget. In order to wake up, you need to tune in, trust, and let it flow.

✿ Try This: Follow Your Feelings

Emotions are called *feelings* because you *feel* them. They hook in, stir up, and move through your body. To follow this natural progression, create some private time and let yourself think of something that infuriates you (politics, the economy, social injustice, a recent insult). Where does this activate your body? What does it feel like, look like, and sound like? Feelings of anger can tighten your jaw, send spikes of energy down your arms, and sound like a low growl. Now think of something profoundly sad. Perhaps sadness can feel heavy in your chest, tearful in your eyes, and sound like a soft sigh. Like many people, your emotional expression might be awkward, resistant, or muted. Is it easy to give voice to that growl or sigh? Can your arms find an appropriate gesture to express anger or sadness?

If emotions are stuck, tucked, and stored in your body, they'll muffle your senses. You know how hard it is to see, hear, or feel clearly when your feelings are triggered. It's also hard to think clearly and make sensible decisions. This is how the past confuses the present and confounds the future. Demystifying your body's emotional process helps you feel more comfortable with your feelings and make sense of the world. As you awaken your emotional body, you may find some emotions more familiar than others. Perhaps some feel nonexistent. Can you access a full spectrum of emotional feeling in your body? Can you express all of your emotions with sounds and gestures? Can you feel where certain emotions live in your body? For instance, you might find the emotional feeling of gratitude (loving, caring) in your chest, and the sound could be a soft *aaah*. It makes it all more manageable if you see your emotions as just another part of your sensitive body. Waking up means emotional intelligence.

Spirit Lives in the Body Too

Seen from the perspective of your body, there wouldn't be life without spirit. When someone is *spirited*, we mean they embody a certain essence that's associated with being vibrant and animated. But even in your quietest moment, spirit is the essential ingredient for being alive. Yet, most people think of spirit as either a philosophical construct or an ephemeral (out of body) experience. Being spiritual is both intimate and personal when you find it living right in your own body. What a gift, then, to discover that your connection to spirit is actually as easy and normal as breathing.

The Latin *spiritu* is the root word for both "respiration" and "spirit." With each breath you take, you become spirit with living. One way to view it is that each cycle of respiration (inhale and exhale) is re-spiriting your body. In this simple, physical context, you actively partake in the miracle of life and connect up with all life. You're in the spaciousness of the present moment. It's not surprising, then, that many spiritual seekers use the breath to help them quiet the mind and be more conscious. And as you've already discovered, focusing on any aspect of your sensual body can quiet your mind and focus your awareness to be in the now. Seeking consciousness is not just for adepts and gurus. It is about waking up and showing up for life at its most mundane, as well as its most sublime. Waking up means showing up—body, mind, and spirit.

Now that you've explored the what, why, where, and how of waking up, you've taken significant steps towards living in an awakened state. Operating on autopilot is no longer an option. Your entire perspective shifted some pages ago when you began to change your mind about your body. If this shifted your idea of who you are and where your body fits in the picture, it's time to use your new perspective and take a fresh look at your health and health care, your relationships and feelings, your strengths and assets, and the meaning of life.

What Is Body Wisdom?

You can be smart without being wise. Waking up is not enough, so where does body wisdom come into the picture? Won't people just get wiser as they get older? Not necessarily. We all know some oldsters that seem pretty out of it and foolish. This is easy to understand from the body's point of view. If you get mired in years and years of negative patterns and pervasive habits (both physical and mental), you're stuck. If you stop moving forward and get set in your ways, life becomes pretty predictable and static. This is both painful and boring. The detritus piles up, rigidity gets entrenched, and you have fewer and fewer options. All of your experience and understanding comes from viewing the horizon from the same perspective. You've stopped growing and exploring your edge.

The first step to getting unstuck is to get moving. Change a pattern, break a habit; do something—anything—differently. Stand up straight and look at the horizon. Instead of plugging into TV or social media, read or just be quiet. Find a positive affirmation and say it each day. Validate your feelings. Take time to be in life and feel some joy. Challenge yourself to take a risk. Change the trajectory and explore the edge a bit. Hey, you've already done a lot of new, edgy things just in reading this first chapter. You've tried things you never thought of before.

The gift of wisdom will be given over time to those who wake up, show up, and stand on the edge—where all growth happens. Your personal edge is where life is examined, wounds are healed, and experience teaches compassion. When you challenge yourself to stand on this edge, your life is an unfolding process where you can say, "Oh, this choice (decision, relationship, or idea) didn't work out so well," "What did my body know [see, feel, or learn]?" and "How can this experience help me be wiser in the future?" As you go through life, being awake means staying current and learning from your mistakes. It also means being true to yourself and your body. It means logging in experience and acting from your heart, as well as your mind. Eventually, you'll come to a place of enlightenment and grace. It is a journey up the mountain that your awakened body, mind, and spirit are taking together.

Just like the wise old man/woman in fairy tales, the face of wisdom is full of scars and lines that tell of a life lived. True wisdom also has a way of perceiving that looks into the soul and sees the eternal journey of humankind looking back.

Two
Body Wisdom IQ Test

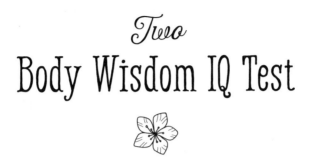

Take this test to see how tuned in you are to your body. Answering the following questions will give you an idea about how much of your body's intelligence you are actually using. After you finish reading *A Guide to Body Wisdom*, it'll be interesting to take a post-test to see just how much your Body Wisdom IQ has increased.

1. What does it feel like when you check in with your body?

    a. It's an unfamiliar or blank space below my head.

    b. It's a collection of various tensions, pains, and sensations.

    c. My body is vibrantly alive and fully present in this moment.

2. What part of your body feels like *you*?

    a. Just my head.

    b. My upper body only, from the waist or chest upward.

    c. My entire body is one integrated, homogenous whole.

3. What is your relationship with tension in your body?

    a. It seems like a normal, nonnegotiable and/or ever-present state.

    b. It gets triggered by external circumstances and feels out of my control.

    c. It can diminish readily when I focus on relaxation and letting go.

4. How do you talk about your posture?

    a. Genetics and bad habits have shaped my posture and there is nothing I can do.

    b. I know about posture and proper mechanics, but it's a constant struggle and disappointment.

    c. I make the connection between posture and outlook and align my posture with my goals.

5. What best describes your relationship with your body?

    a. Boss to subordinate/coach to athlete/driver to car.

    b. Parent to disobedient/spoiled/recalcitrant child.

    c. Respectful companions/partners/allies on the journey of life.

6. What is your internal dialogue?

    a. Talking with my body would be pointless and feel silly.

    b. Demanding/dismissive/critical, mostly one-way.

    c. Positive self-talk is very important and, in return, I listen to my body.

7. When you're engaged in routine physical activity (eating a meal, brushing your hair, cleaning house, exercising) do you

    a. blank out, proceed robotically, or multitask?

    b. find yourself berating or complaining about your body being too smelly, slow, fat, clumsy, not good enough?

    c. encourage yourself with positive slogans and invite gracefulness into the most menial of tasks?

8. Do you know how each part of your body functions and what your body needs in order to function well?

    a. I turn all of this responsibility over to my doctor.

    b. I am learning as I go along. If something breaks down, I get information and help to correct the problem.

c. I am fascinated by how my body works and seek the latest information to help understand and take good care of it.

9. Do you feel your tissues, bones, and organs?

   a. It's all a mystery to me.

   b. I feel connected to my body in general but can't differentiate individual parts.

   c. My sensory awareness includes my organs, bones, and muscles. This is part of my feedback loop between body and mind.

10. When you awaken from sleep, do you

    a. struggle to wake up or wish you could slumber forever?

    b. need to use your willpower to propel your body out of bed?

    c. take some time to feel the day, move your fingers and toes and say a few words of gratitude before your body begins its active day?

11. When you go to sleep, do you

    a. need to use alcohol, drugs, or TV in order to relax?

    b. push your body to a point of exhaustion and simply pass out?

    c. take some time to finish your day, quiet your mind, and relax your body?

12. How do you handle fatigue or illness?

    a. I'm impatient and override my feelings, proceeding with business as usual.

    b. I modify my plans accordingly, cut myself some slack, and take steps to bolster my immune system.

    c. I become proactive and proceed as a wise, loving steward of my body. I take measures and give positive messages to set the course for a return to robust health.

13. Do you think your thoughts influence your physical body?

    a. Such beliefs are magical thinking/pseudoscience/a bunch of hogwash.

    b. I do self-improvement mantras/positive affirmations and think its my fault when health and performance aren't top-notch.

    c. Being mindful of my thoughts is an important way to make sure my body is healthy and happy.

14. Are you seeking balanced activity in your daily routines?

    a. I'm too busy to play and the only time I rest is when I am sleeping.

    b. I play hard and work hard; I rest when I can do no more.

    c. I challenge myself to identify old habits and recalibrate so work/play/rest are balanced each day.

15. How do your emotions live in your body?

    a. It's upsetting to think about my feelings and generally my body feels pretty numb.

    b. I work hard to control my feelings but periodically they rear their ugly head and spin out of control.

    c. When I respond to my emotions like a form of poetry, I'm comfortable and responsible with their expression.

16. How is it for you when you're alone in nature?

    a. It never happens. Whenever it happens, I'm uncomfortable and can't wait to get home.

    b. My mind is on a nonstop rollercoaster ride of distracting thoughts and uncomfortable feelings.

    c. It feels natural to be in nature. It's a source of replenishment and comfort.

17. What is your experience of physical intimacy?

    a. I hate to be touched/I'm always horny/I do everything I can to avoid it.

b. My memories, distractions, and judgments get in the way unless I use alcohol, drugs, or porn.

c. My body is the conduit for the distinct pleasure and nonverbal experience of love and passion. My positive self-consciousness gives me many nuanced and creative ways to express myself in a wide range of intimate situations.

18. How have you commemorated the significant passages in your life (puberty, graduations, birthdays, losses, healing, moving, etc.)?

a. They're no big deal; they come and go.

b. I'm squirmy and uncomfortable with any fuss, so intentionally avoid anything personal or celebratory.

c. Ceremony and ritual (traditional, as well as personal) have marked many passages and helped me move on to the next chapter. They enrich my life.

19. How do you feel about body functions and conditions that feel out of your control (allergies, acne, moles, freckles, eczema, wrinkles, as well as digestive processes, menstruation, orgasm, sweat, tears, goose bumps, blushing, and fluids such as blood, mucous, semen, discharge)?

a. All of this is unseemly and simply an unfortunate part of having a body.

b. I take care of the problems and endure the rest.

c. It's all kind of fascinating, a part of being alive.

20. How do you feel about your body when it needs extra care or healing (digestive imbalance, sexual function, overuse injuries, chronic or acute conditions)?

a. It makes me angry (disgusted, confused, depressed, scared) and I want it to all go away.

b. I feel anxious and isolated, wanting someone else to take over (health professional, mother/father, god).

c. I take this as a wake-up call and opportunity to learn more about my body. Although I have no problem asking for help, I know my body is a vital partner in the healing process.

21. How do you think or talk about your death?

a. I don't. To me, the topic is morbid and creepy.

b. I've made peace with it, taken care of the legalities, but it makes me uncomfortable to talk about it.

c. This is as important and connected to life as birth. I have conveyed my thoughts to loved ones about end-of-life issues and, when it comes, I'll look forward to the great mystery.

Simply taking the Body Wisdom IQ test gets you in touch with your body and invites your curious mind to wonder "why"? Although the answers might not nail your attitudes and feelings exactly, you get the gist. Now, it's time to score the test and see how you did. Then, read on. Many of these areas of *body intelligence* will be discussed and explored in the following chapters.

Scoring

You will accrue 1, 2, or 3 points depending on your answer to each question. For example, **a=1**; **b=2**; and **c=3**. Add all of these to determine your score on the Body Wisdom IQ scale.

0 to 21 points: This book will surprise you and introduce you to your body as a brand new source of intelligence and awareness. Reading *A Guide to Body Wisdom* will change your life. It may save your life.

22 to 42 points: As you continue your pursuit of a full, healthy, and happy life, this book will help you find, understand and utilize your body's innate assets. The information and experiences will add to what you know so you can cultivate and enjoy life to the fullest.

43 to 63 points: This book will affirm what you already know and delight you with some new information, perspectives, and ideas for living in your conscious, smart body. It will offer you many ways to find a deep and abiding wisdom. As a constant reference source, *A Guide to Body Wisdom* will be the book you give to your family and friends.

Three
The Basics

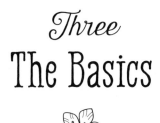

Once you wake up and learn to trust your smart body, it's time to design a basic self-care program that really works. When you know how to listen, your body can help you evaluate what you need, what works, and what doesn't. When you don't know how to listen, figuring out what to do can be confusing and overwhelming. This chapter will introduce you to your body's basic needs and help you find the way to optimal health.

Like most people, you probably brush, bathe, eat, and sleep as a matter of routine and hardly give much thought to how you care for your body. It's only when you want it to conform, perform, or stop complaining that you stop to wonder if something's missing. Then when you decide to be proactive and get some information, you run into a daunting cascade of conflicting facts and opinions about diet, exercise, sleep, and lifestyle. It's difficult to know what to do or if you're on the right track. Let this book help you start at the beginning and reconfigure your basic body care. Regardless of your health or fitness profile, tending to the basics will reboot your enthusiasm and get you on the path to radiant health and happiness. From the perspective of your body, it's easier to take ownership of a self-care regimen when it makes sense.

❋ Try This: Trust Your Body

To identify what you need and implement an inspired self-care program, you'll need to get to know and begin to trust your body. Use your awake body as a personal compass or GPS, and let it help you zero in on your deepest truth. If you're uncertain about what course to take or decision to make, why not listen to your body and let it lead the way? Each time you encounter a suggestion or an exercise in this book, check in with your body and invite its input. Try on the basic care elements in this chapter (and throughout this book) as if they were clothing. Ask your body, "Does this fit, or not?" If your body stays open and comfortable while exploring the various activities and protocols, it's probably telling you, "Yes, I am ready for this now," or "This matches my needs." If you feel your body contract, pull back, or stop breathing, perhaps it is saying "No, let's hold off on this one for a bit." Quite simply, whenever your body gives you the nod, go ahead and try it out. If not, trust yourself and move on. Putting your body to work as a sounding board will both customize your experience and make sure that you're getting the specific help you need. As you learn to trust your body, it will begin to trust you! Why not start today?

Of course, you've been taking care of your body. You've been brushing your teeth (flossing?) and feeding yourself (on the run?) and washing (power shower?) for years. Yet, like most people in this stress-ridden, achievement-driven culture, taking really good care of your body is a hit or miss sort of thing. Take a moment now to consider your personal relationship to some of these body basics:

- **Skin care:** Does exfoliating, moisturizing, or massaging feel like an indulgence?

- **Moving:** Does exercise or taking a walk feel like another chore?

- **Food:** Does a sensible diet bring up emotion or resistance?

- **Play:** Is finding time for play one of the core elements of your lifestyle or does your recreation feel like work?

- **Relaxation:** Do you create time each day for leisure or is high gear your only speed?

- **Sleep:** Do you prepare for sleep or expect it just to happen and get frustrated when it doesn't?

- **Aesthetics:** Are you aware of the appearance/feel/pleasure of your living/working space? Does it reflect a sense of design, proportion, and beauty, as well as function and efficiency?

When your body counts, these questions have a new meaning. Doing something about the answers will improve every aspect of your life. Setting up the basics of self-care creates the very foundation for your quality of life: how you relate, how you communicate, how you inspire, how you create, how you love, and how you heal. Even if you're suffering from years of neglect, illness, injury, or overuse, you can be a powerful catalyst for change right now just by getting in touch with your body wisdom. No matter where you start, taking care of your body will save you a lot of grief, time, and energy. It may even salvage your dreams for the future.

Jim. Jim had a lifelong dream of surfing around the world. For many years, rest and exercise were low priority as his business and family thrived. In his stressful schedule there was rarely a moment when he wasn't on the go. Sure, he would find time to be in the ocean when the surf was up, but he never had time to do the stretching and toning his body needed to prepare for the sport. His motto was "If it ain't broke, don't fix it." Over time, Jim's self-care profile started to show the results and his body lost its resiliency. The combination of stress and neglect eventually contributed to a serious shoulder injury and turned his dream into a disappointing nightmare. The motto might have worked for an automobile, but it certainly didn't work for his body. He needed his body to transport him to all of his dreams and he couldn't trade it in. In order to heal, Jim needed to put his body front and center in his priorities. Seeking expert advice and listening to his body helped him get into low gear to do the necessary rehab. Not only did Jim's shoulder heal and regain its strength, but when he took his smart body surfing, he was even better at his sport.

As Jim discovered, it's not prudent to compromise your body care now for some reward in the future. Much as you'd like, you can't trade up for a new model. This is your vehicle for the whole ride. The choices you make right now can set a trajectory for vitality, resiliency, stamina, and happiness into the future. At any given point, you're either moving toward health and balance or you're not. Tend to your basics and your health dividends will accrue like money in the bank.

Taking Stock

You've been taking care of yourself for many years. Over time you've probably learned a fair amount about what works and what doesn't. Each time you encountered an injury, illness, change, or challenge, you had an opportunity to find out more about your body and fine-tune your self-care. Even with the guidance of health experts, some of the most important things you know came through the experience of trial and error. It's helpful to think of your body and its ongoing care as a puzzle with some of the pieces in flux. To take stock of what's in place, what's missing, and what's needed, bring along your personal experience and start where you are now. Like anyone on a journey, you may be cruising along in good health with no complaints. You may be slogging through the mud unable to get traction or make progress. You may be stuck and stymied at a hurdle or roadblock. You may feel as if you're careening on a wild ride into the unknown. Even if you're cruising, you'll learn something about yourself when you ask your body, "What is missing?" and "What do you need?" Give your body a say in the discussion and it will help you understand the fine print in your owner's manual.

✿ Explore: Your Personal Health Profile

Get out your Body Wisdom journal and compile a few notes to help you take a good look at your health profile. This is more about awareness than a recantation of your health history. Take some time to check in and ask what your body thinks. Answering the following prompts will ensure you've covered the basics.

Consider your flesh and bones.

Do you have the strength and flexibility that you want/need? Can you touch your toes and walk up a steep hill? Are you accommodating a long-term injury or chronic weakness? Do you take time to exercise aerobically? What is the condition of the skin on your arms and legs, as well as your face?

Consider your organs and glands.

Do you have the energy you need? Does the food you eat give you high-grade fuel? Are you easily startled and/or often anxious? Can you find your calm center whenever you need it? Do your eyes look bright and alert? Does your facial expression appear unhappy, fatigued, or depleted?

Consider your attitude.

Are you focused and peaceful when attending to your body's needs? Do you value the time spent brushing, bathing, feeding, stretching, and so on as a part of the quality of life? Do you enjoy being physical—moving, dancing, bathing, working, touching, and loving?

Consider your balance.

Are you resilient and responsive to change? Do you get the rest you need? Does your schedule have time set aside for play? Does your demeanor communicate love and hope? When you see a photo of yourself, do you see worry and stress?

Jot down everything that comes to mind in your journal. Write a brief summary and let it all rest for a day or two. When you reread your notes, see them from the perspective of a health analyst and evaluate your personal health profile. This will give you a good idea of where you are now and what you need to do in order to tend to the basics. Jot your diagnosis and prescription for what's lacking and what's needed. Keep these notes to refer to later on. Committing to just one suggestion from this chapter will influence your health profile over time. Like any course correction, when you change the slightest thing, you shift the whole trajectory.

A Guide to Body Wisdom is not about one particular program or philosophy. Many experts can tell you about the necessity and protocols of good breathing, eating, exercise, and sleep. This book puts your smart body front and center where it belongs. Take that leap of faith—trust your body to show you where you need to start, what you need to know, and how to access your own authority. When you tune in to the flesh and bones of your body, the basics will make sense and self-care will be personalized and sustainable.

Breathing

As a function of the autonomic nervous system, your breathing happens on its own, but full and efficient breaths can be hindered by structural holding patterns and long-term habits. Of course you're breathing, but are you breathing well? Does your inhale and exhale flow freely and fully, without any tension or restriction? Finding and cultivating a familiarity with the free, full, and focused function of respiration is what basic breathing is all about.

✾ *Try This: How's Your Breathing?*

Let's see how your body breathes and establish a baseline to work from. In order to focus your attention inwardly, you'll need to exit the madding crowd. Place this book in your lap, tune in to your interior body-space, and focus on your breathing. Notice what moves (and doesn't move) as you inhale and exhale. The anatomy of a full breath (through the motion initiated by the diaphragm's contraction/release) includes every moving part of your body. If your ribs (spine, pelvis, arms, and legs) aren't also breathing, you have some basic work to do.

If your breathing is restricted in any way, habit and history may be the culprits. How could this happen? Whenever your body encounters something physically or emotionally challenging, it naturally braces and holds on a bit. Just think of what happens to your breath when you're faced with a tense situation, concentrated effort, or unexpected event. Your breath goes on hold a bit, yes? Unless you consciously reset, when the moment passes and circumstances change, your breath will continue to hold on … for hours or even years to come. One of the first things I address when clients come to me is the way their breathing patterns reflect the past rather than the present. Understandably, if you don't have an experiential reference for good breathing, limited breathing can become cumulative, habitual, and just feel normal. Basic breathing is letting anatomy teach you about your full potential.

✾ *Try This: A Basic Breathing Lesson*

To feel the fullness of breath, you'll need to get comfortable, be quiet, and focus on your anatomy. It helps to close your eyes and use your body sense to feel how your ribs move as you exhale and inhale. Do you feel your ribs expand with the in breath and collapse with the out breath? See if you can let go a little more (exhale, relax, release). Then, let your ribs move easily as the air moves in (inhale, expand, release). Basic breathing in this way will help you let go of tension/stress and relax. Now, see if you can feel some of the movement in other places in your body (i.e., your shoulders, collarbone, belly, pelvis, arms/legs, and fingers/toes. If you put your hands on your belly (collarbone, pelvis), can you feel the movement come through? Your breath is a metaphor for life and how you breathe can give you something to ponder beyond simple anatomy. Don't be surprised if your breathing program includes emotional release or spiritual insight (learn more about this in the chapters to come).

Although breathing feels so basic and automatic, most people just aren't good at it. When you begin to address your body's basic needs, breathing is at the top of the list. Learning to breathe well and fully is an ongoing process and a key part of your personal healing. Give it time. It's possible that your functional holding pattern goes back to the very first breath you took and may involve elements of your emotional and physical history that need time to heal. To breathe easily in an unobstructed, conscious way is a lifelong exploration. Practice full breathing every day to unravel the past, be in the present, and give yourself a centered reference point when you get highjacked by the various traumas and dramas of life. Even though breathing seems so very basic, don't hesitate to ask for help. Pilates, yoga, meditation/relaxation, massage/bodywork, and psychotherapy can get things moving when a lifetime of habit has become structural limitation. Breathing well is as essential to your happiness as it is to your health.

Darcy. Darcy took breathing for granted. Even though he often found himself holding his breath, he didn't think it mattered and certainly never wondered why. As we worked together to release his tense muscles, Darcy's attention was directed over and over again to his breathing. No amount of expert bodywork would dislodge the muscular tension in his hips until his ribs let go! Seeing the potential connection, Darcy decided to observe his breathing at random times throughout the day. When he caught himself holding his breath, he asked his body why, and the word fear *popped into his head. It felt as if he was unsure of his balance, much like a toddler learning to walk. It was as if Darcy was stuck at a developmental stage and needed to learn how to walk and breathe at the same time. It may seem obvious, but practicing his walking breath not only freed up his inhale, but helped Darcy feel more balanced and sure of himself.*

Breathing well keeps your body healthy—cells oxygenated, waste products processed, and physiology calmed. It also helps you be calm and stay in the here and now. For this reason, this book will often refer to your breathing body for help.

Eating

How you eat can be as important as *what* you eat. Regardless of the nutrients in any meal, if you consume food in a state of distress or gulp it down on the run, your basic nutrient requirements will not be met. Basic food is about sustenance *and* sensuality. Studies have shown that your digestion and absorption has everything to do with physiology (your body) and psychology (your mind). The way you feel and think when you eat influences the outcome. For instance, if you spend more time chewing, you'll simply absorb more nutrients and register more sensual satisfaction. Being aware when you're eating will change your relationship to food. Here are some ways to take a fresh look at *how* you eat:

- Are you aware of your body's presence and posture?

- Is your mind focused on the food and the moment?

- Does your body have the comfort and time it needs to eat?

- Do you savor and chew your food with full sensory awareness?

- Do you pause at the beginning/end of a meal to be mindful (notice the colors and presentation, give thanks, feel gratitude)?

Perhaps, looking at how you eat is more about you and your body than about the actual food. By this time, you've established a complex, unconscious relationship with eating. Changing how you eat is a powerful catalyst for re-evaluating and bringing your relationship with food up to date.

✳ *Explore: Observe the Meal*

For the next few days, follow these basic eating suggestions for at least one meal a day:

- Serve your meal in a calm and comfortable setting.

- Arrange the food/table with symmetry and beauty.

- Sit facing your food, squarely on the chair.

- Breathe a bit before you commence.

- Notice the food on your plate and be grateful for its nourishment.

- Let your fork rest between bites.

- Chew thoroughly.

- Savor your food—feel the sensation and movement in your jaw, tongue, and throat.

- Pause at the completion of your meal and direct a centering breath to your belly before you leave the table.

Pay attention to how your body and mind experience mealtime. What happens when you eat? This is truly an exercise in mindfulness. After each meal, jot down a few observations in your Body Wisdom journal. Don't worry about diet or nutrition, just observe what's happening with your body. At the same time, be honest with what's floating through your mind. Be cognizant of any self-talk and/or resistance. Connect with your emotions and what might be triggered from old mealtime memories. Give yourself credit for any success and, without judgment, notice when habit overrides conscious intention. Let your curious mind invite insight and encourage awareness rather than perfection. Write it all down. The above protocol sets the stage for a good basic eating practice. This is something to return to over and over whenever it feels like you've gotten off track with good eating habits.

You might be startled at what pops up when you observe your meals. There's no doubt about it, the way you eat now can be traced right back to your emotional history. In order to show up for mealtime, you might need to change an old mindset. Here are some memories and attitudes that were uncovered when Judy, Shane, and Pamela paid attention to mealtime:

- Judy felt that eating was just another chore. She would've loved to find a nutritional pill that would free her from the prep and ceremony of mealtime.

- Shane's memories of being grilled and criticized as a child came up every time he sat down at the table. He preferred to eat and exit as quickly as possible.

- Pamela approached preparing, serving, and enjoying a meal simply as a way of life. She felt disappointed and lonely when her tablemates didn't share her enthusiasm.

In order to show up without preconceived ideas and expectations, these folks needed to unhook their emotions from the past. Perhaps when Judy gives herself time for sensuality, Shane separates his emotions from his food, and Pamela lets go of expectations, their new mind-sets will let them show up 100 percent for mealtime, present-time.

Looking at how you eat can be about more than fork, knife, and food. Like Judy, Shane, and Pamela realized, how you eat is determined by how you think and feel. How you feed yourself can also reflect how well you nurture yourself.

Lorrie. As a high-powered casting director, Lorrie was always multitasking with no time to spare. Not only did she eat on the run, she felt as if she bathed, slept, and made love on the run as well. When she took the challenge to observe her meals, she was shocked to see herself standing up and gulping down her food as if there would never be enough. Slowing down for self-reflection, Lorrie saw how her way of eating (and working) was linked to her fear of scarcity. For her Little Self, there would never be enough time, energy, money, or food. Curiously, when Lorrie made herself simply sit at the table, not only did her basic way of eating change but she started to feel "fed" creatively, emotionally, and financially as well.

When you focus on how you eat, you're bound to run into your relationship with food. Just like you learned in the previous chapter, your relationship with food will lighten up when you stop judging/bossing/chastising your body and start trusting it. When your relationship to food changes, what/how much/why you eat changes along with it. It's a natural progression. Let your wise body lead you to the foods that feel good and work for you. Listen to your wise body when it tells you when and how much to eat. Basic eating means more than surviving, it also means thriving. Along with basic breathing, it's a foundation piece for body wisdom.

Moving

Your body mechanics were designed to allow you to run, jump, curl up in a ball, tie your shoes, throw a Frisbee, and so much more. One of nature's sassy laws applies to you: "If you don't move it, you lose it." This is how it goes—if you don't use your body's full range of motion, a habit of limitation becomes a holding pattern, and holding patterns get set and limit your range of motion over time. When you pay attention to your body as it executes the simplest task, you may be surprised by how little you actually move. Instead of using your whole body to scoop down and pick up a pencil from the floor, you brace and strain to pick it up with your fingertips. Instead of using your whole body to carry a suitcase, you brace and clutch it with your hand and arm. Did you know that any time you abbreviate movement or isolate a workload, you're making things harder, not easier?

Most people never learned how to move fully or efficiently and simply took on the habits of those around them. Sometimes, movement patterns were further limited when injury occurred and compensation left them unable to regain full function. Is your past inhibiting your body's ability to move as it was designed? Get in touch with your basic movement patterns and begin to untangle old compensations as well as years of habit. When I taught my Moving With Ease class, many people came with muscular aches and pains directly related to bad movement habits. Isabel had carpal tunnel syndrome because she typed with her arms and wrists taut while her fingers pounded away. Rocco had chronic tension in his shoulders and neck from clutching the steering wheel. Anne had sciatica due to running while the rest of her body was on hold. Whether typing, driving, or running, part of their bodies moved while the rest was braced and tight. Is there any discomfort you have that might need to move a little more? To repair the aches/pains and establish good movement hygiene, you need to call on some basic movement wisdom in order to become mechanically whole again. Whether doing something small like brushing your hair or something big like climbing Denali, your mechanical body moves best if you don't hold it back.

❀ Try This: Movement Matters

Feel the effect of body mechanics on energy expenditure. Without changing your position, hold this book out in front of you for ten seconds. Feel your muscle effort and register the weightiness of the book as the seconds tick by. Return to your starting position, shake out your arms, and try it again. This time, however, use your whole body and let your pelvis pivot to bring your ribs, shoulder, and arm forward together as you lift the book. This way, your body works as a mechanical whole instead of isolated parts. What's the difference? Does it seem easier when you use your whole body? Does the book seem lighter? Your body was designed to make moving easy. See if you can replicate this experience in other activities, such as lifting and carrying a grocery bag, doing house and garden work, or brushing your hair and teeth.

❀ Try This: How Does Your Body Move?

Pay attention to how your body moves for the next few days. Break down the experience and feel how the segments of your body (feet, legs, hips, et cetera) participate as you lean over to pick up something from the floor, reach out for a handshake, or do any mundane, normal task. Be aware of the range of motion in your bones and joints. Does it feel as if the simplest movement is abbreviated and held back? Could this be habit or structure? Do you use your whole body or minimize movement? Does your body feel fluid or stuck? Your body needs to move and to move well in order to be healthy and happy. Now, see how your range and ease of motion change when you use your whole body. You might feel self-conscious and a bit clumsy at first, but just think of it as the dance of loading groceries into the car, folding the laundry, or picking up your clothes.

Get Your Moves Down.

All physical activity has a basic movement component, even if it seems hardly physical. Even when you're still, your breathing ribs are still moving. No matter what you're doing, your body will be at ease all day/night long if you release your holding pattern to move more freely again. Since holding patterns are entrenched and reinforced through lack of awareness and habit, you'll need to pay attention and practice. Here are some good times to practice full-body, integrated moving:

- When you walk to work, let your hips and arms swing naturally and your head and neck move freely.

- When you brush your hair, feel the pressure on your feet shift with the motion above.

- When you work out at the gym, feel the strength come from the core and the effort coordinated throughout your body. Choose workouts that use your whole body rather than isolated parts.

- When you wipe the countertop (or wash the car, paint a wall, or mow the lawn), let the action include all of your body.

It might help to exaggerate a bit to get the hang of it, but don't mistake full-body movement with random flailing or over-movement. Basic movement is sensible and appropriate. It is also calibrated precisely for each activity. After all, when you take a sip of water, you don't want the gesture to be so dramatic that you spill all over yourself! Your goal is to explore the purely mechanical nature of any given activity. For instance, your hips, knees, and ankles naturally transfer weight forward to the front of your foot when you pick up something from the floor; when you're walking, your head bobs slightly. From the mundane to the artistic, basic movement includes your whole body—from the base of your feet to the top of your head. If your movement is restricted, your body will feel braced and overworked. If your movement is fluid, your body will feel enlivened. When you stop resisting and start respecting your body's mechanical design, every movement you make will be efficient and pleasing. The most arduous work is graceful; the most tedious task, a dance.

Metaphorically, it's easy to see how being stuck, rigid, or braced can influence your self-image and what you project to others. You can learn a lot about yourself (and others) by observing how your body moves. If your attitude about life is optimistic and confident, you'll feel exuberant and enlivened as you move. If your attitude is defeated or stagnant, you'll feel stiff and tired as you move. Or, maybe, you feel depressed *because* your movements are repressed. When you pause to observe your moving body, the connection between physical and emotional might surprise you. Could it be that your hesitant, stuck body is actually holding an expression of the past?

Paying attention to how you move can help you shift things around and bring everything up to date. Imagine that your walking body represents this metaphor: You walk forward into the future, not backward into the past. From your body's point of view, anything that is riveted in the past gets left behind when you take that step into the future. Your walking body gets you going again anytime you feel off kilter, burdened, uninspired, or unaware. It helps you move beyond limitation and hesitation. Tune in to your body mechanics and free your full potential. Let your moving body be poetry in motion.

Hank. Through his tai chi practice, Hank was able to explore his reticence and find his personal power. In the beginning he felt self-conscious and ineffective doing the reaching/punching movements. His arms seemed to pull back instead of pushing forward to complete the gestures gracefully. This reminded him of how in life, he felt diminished and was afraid to be seen. As old memories of teasing and torment flooded forth, his tai chi gave him the opportunity to reframe the wounds—symbolically reaching beyond his limitations and punching through resistance. Freeing up his moving body helped him heal the past and claim his future. Rather than pulling back from his talents and opportunities, Hank felt empowered to reach out.

Fitness

It's a natural segue from basic movement to basic fitness. To be fit, your body needs to move well. In order to move well your body needs to be strong and limber. Basic fitness requires an exercise routine of some sort and a mindset. Getting your body and mind aligned with basic fitness is a very personal, ongoing, day-by-day process. Whether exercising is a way of life or a recurring frustration, taking a fresh look from the perspective of your smart body will invite something new to the conversation.

Whether or not you're well versed in the dos and don'ts of exercise, approaching fitness from your body's perspective will help you find and design a route to fitness that's both personalized and inspired. In order to help your mind and body take a fresh look, consider the following:

- Do you vacillate between being in shape and being out of shape?

- What is your relationship to exercise? How do you really feel about it?

- Is your body an equal partner or is your mind the dominant one?

- What self-talk or attitude motivates you?

- What self-talk or attitude gets in your way?

- What is your present commitment?
  - Are you consistent?
  - Do you show up 100 percent?
  - Are you getting the results you want?

Then notice how you felt when you considered these questions. Did you feel encouraged or rewarded, defeated or chastised? Taking a fresh look means just that. It's not about getting discouraged, defensive, or self-judgmental—those attitudes are history. Let go of old assumptions and emotional frustrations. Your fresh look is a fresh start.

You need your body *and* your mind to be on board and inspired for fitness. When you take a fresh look, your smart mind can identify old habits of laziness and emotional overlays. For instance, just because you've spent most of your life avoiding exercise doesn't mean your body won't benefit from sweating; just because your gut clenches at the thought of joining a softball league doesn't mean you won't have fun once you move beyond your fear of rejection; just because your body feels agitated doesn't mean it needs a sedative; just because you're tired doesn't mean you need to rest; and just because you've managed your anger by taking it for a run doesn't mean this is a good idea. Your mind is savvy to the physiological ramifications and psychological complexities of exercise. Let it help you decipher the mixed messages from the real deal. Once you've sorted through the "what ifs" and "yes buts," your smart mind can sit in the director's chair and help you pursue a fitness program that really works.

Let your smart body be in charge of feedback. It can tell you what works, what needs to be done, and what progress you're making. It also gives you perks and rewards. In addition to strength and resiliency, the return on your efforts will include improved vitality, mood, sleep, digestion, and mental acuity. Your body will also let you know if you're on the wrong track. You can count on it to let you know (sometimes, not so pleasantly) when you push too hard, stretch too long, slack off, or lack respect. Running the same old and tired routines of bribing, bossing, punishing, and shaming is no way to treat your body, and it doesn't work.

❀ Explore: Be Your Inner Trainer

Exercising is a very personal deal. You're the one spinning on the bicycle, holding the yoga pose, pumping uphill on the hiking trail. Hard, challenging work is the perfect time to check out your self-talk and align it with your fitness goals. Not only does your body hear what you're saying, it believes it. When you learn to coach your body with respect and positive encouragement, your body responds accordingly.

Over the next week, no matter where you are on the fitness scale, listen to yourself. Do what you do, but do some kind of exercise each day and listen to yourself. Your first task as the Inner Trainer is to ferret out and reframe unproductive attitudes and self-talk. Make a list of these in your Body Wisdom journal and creatively morph each negative into a positive, allowing your interior dialogue to participate in your success! Ask yourself the following:

- Am I hearing old ideas and judgments from the past?

- Is this my original script or did it come from somewhere else?

- Does my self-talk sound friendly, encouraging, and patient?

- How does this make me feel?

Before you can think clearly about where you want to be and how you're going to get there, you may need to jettison some old baggage. It's simple: hear the words and feel the feelings; then, change the words and change the feelings; writing it all down and highlighting your new affirmations. The discipline you need right now is one of blunt honesty and zero tolerance. After all, you don't want your words and attitudes to undermine your commitment before you even start.

George. George listened to podcasts while he exercised on the elliptical machine every morning and paid attention to everything else in the world except his body. So, when he decided to take a fresh look, he turned off the news and listened to his body for a week. When it was just George and his body alone at the workout, he was dismayed to hear the undercurrent of self-criticism in his "personal podcast." He prodded his body with taunts such as, "Come on, lard butt," and "Get the lead out," or "Let it burn." These were phrases he hadn't consciously heard since grade school, but they felt as hurtful now as they did then. As his own Inner Trainer, George needed to replace these words with something truly helpful like, "I feel my legs and they feel good," or "Breathing hard helps my lungs and my heart." Such simple appreciation for his body shifted his vision from the past to the future AND made the workout feel more playful.

Coco. Coco set a goal of running for an extra fifteen minutes. When she pushed past her usual time on the track, she was surprised to hear the sound of self-sabotage. Knowing the importance of being positive, it was unsettling to hear her inner assessment: "What's the use anyway? I'll never be any good." Of course, these words felt like carrying a load of bricks on her back. Rooting out the source for her pessimism, she recalled her dad saying, "'Pretty good' isn't worth a damn." She remembered feeling discouraged before even giving anything a try. Setting her own standard for success, Coco decided to change the words to "'Pretty good' is pretty damned good."

Remember: Your body has feelings and needs respect. When your body and mind are on the same fitness program, your words and actions confirm that your efforts are respected, encouraged, and recognized. As a team, your body and mind enhance the success of any fitness goal.

Set Up Success

Once you get your mind and body on the same team, you're ready to set up a successful fitness program. Start where you are now, give yourself a challenge, and build to where you want to be. For some people this might be doing the stairs at work and getting out of breath. Others might add a few reps in the weight room or take a dance class or hike with a friend twice a week. What you choose to do is less important than being consistent and conscious. Following are some general guidelines for success:

- Set aside time in your schedule that is nonnegotiable.

- Choose exercise that is pleasing and appropriate for your age, current ability, and body type.

- Include elements of stretching, toning, loosening, and breathing hard/sweating.

- Start where you are now and build slowly over time.

- Make sure you visit your full range and maximum effort—build it up and wind it down—in each session.

- When you exercise, get into your body (music is okay, but television, podcasts, reading, fantasizing, processing feelings, and so forth will take you out of your body).

- See this as a process, *not* a project.

No matter what works for you, how you *think* sets your body up for success or failure. This is not simply mind over matter—basic fitness is all about mind with matter! Having a body-centered statement to fuel your commitment is the perfect way to get yourself going.

✿ Try This: Your Body-Powered Statement

Find a positive phrase to change your attitude about fitness and motivate your good intentions. The idea is to find the magic words that will help your body wake up and remember its original design for moving, working, breathing, and sweating. To find the body-powered statement that works for you, close your eyes and imagine your body moving and exercising with strength, stamina, and flexibility. Visualize your body embracing *fitness* fully and exuberantly. Use this picture to construct a motivational mantra that's body powered. Some good ones:

- "My body is designed to be strong and flexible."

- "Being fit and vital is being alive."

- "Little by little, day by day, my body's getting fit."

- "I'm body-conscious rather than self-conscious."

- "I'm training for my sport and my sport is life."

You could also find the exact message that works for you to ameliorate your resistance and judgment. Write your body-powered statement on a Post-it and put it where you'll see it (bathroom mirror, message board, refrigerator, dashboard). Let this motivational mantra become your new self-talk. Repeat it over and over as you exercise or drive, brush your teeth, and so on. Now when you listen to yourself, you'll hear a positive message that aligns your body with your commitment.

Look a Little Deeper

Tending to your basic fitness is a personal journey. What works for you won't necessarily work for someone else. Socially, the subject of fitness and exercise is a loaded topic, and everyone has something to say. Bring it up over coffee or at a dinner party and watch what happens. You'll hear opinions, facts, projections, and conjectures. But if the conversation turns to personal experience, the attention of the group will fragment because, well, it's just too personal. Like brushing your teeth or washing between your toes, tending to basic fitness is one of your most intimate assignments. Stretched over the course of your lifetime, it's more of an ongoing process than a specific program. As George and Coco discovered in the examples earlier, this process can uncover some emotional history.

Getting your body moving can get your emotions moving. Instead of getting blindsided, just let this be part of the process. Because your body can hold your personal story, worries, fears, disappointments, regrets, and traumas, simply moving around has the potential for healing. If some rotten old ideas and festering feelings float to the top, trust your wise body to move the sludge out of your body *and* your psyche. Your personal circumstances are tailor-made for growth and healing. See how Gayle, Pattie, and Tom found a key to process some emotional residue when they tended to basic fitness, and check out chapter 6: The Emotional Body, for a deeper look.

Gayle. Gayle needed to change her mind about her body. Taking care of herself was a low priority, including any basic fitness needs. She vowed to get around to it once she had her finances in order, her employment issues resolved, and her daughter's health problems were under control. Months stretched to years, her weight went up, her vitality went down, and Gayle found herself frustrated by her bad habits. One day, she heard a podcast that inspired her to take a look at the past in order to get a grip on the present. Both her mom and dad were in the hospitality business and often the needs of others took priority over the family. Gayle could recognize this same pattern in her life. To make the time to get to the gym, she needed to listen to her personal needs for herself alone. From this place, she could devise and commit to a fitness program that had meaning. It wasn't long before she had the epiphany that taking care of her own needs first was the only way to show up for others.

Pattie. Pattie wanted to look good and used her mind to drive her fitness. She pushed herself hard, and when her body complained, she simply increased her willpower. For her, it was mind over matter every time even when her body really needed help. Approaching fitness from the outside short-circuited messages from the inside and ended up compromising the very fitness she revered. As pain turned into numbness and disability, Pattie finally sought medical help and discovered she had a tumor that needed immediate surgery. Her physical situation was a wake-up call, and Pattie used her recovery time to "surgically" remove the idea that how she looked was more important than how she felt. Now she realized she needed to love her body into healing. Pattie's new mantra, "It all comes from the inside," allowed her to be able to exercise in order to feel good… and look good.

Tom. Tom managed such a truckload of personal history that his creativity was backed into a corner and his health was constantly breaking down. Instead of being able to move forward in his life, he was frozen in his tracks. His emotions and thoughts were shackled by acrid memories and the future seemed like an uphill climb. Tom's therapist urged him to take a chance on his body and move against resistance. Following the wise slogan, "the only place to start is where you are," he took a short walk each day down to the mailbox at the end of his road. Over time, as his walk lengthened to a stroll around the neighborhood, Tom imagined he was moving away from the restriction of the past and toward the potential of the future. Rather than sit around and rust with inactivity, his body got moving, his gears greased up, and his load lightened up. Going slowly let the old pictures and postures steadily melt away. Tom's next slogan became, "I am renewed with each step I take."

Looking deeper at some of your personal issues will clear the way so your commitment to fitness can get going and be successful. Like many people, you may need to excavate some crusty old ideas and refresh them with positive intentions. Your personal history has shaped your view. Once you see the picture more clearly, you can revise the image, find a motivational slogan, and rewrite the script. As you know from the previous chapter, what you say leaves an impression and sets the stage. So pay attention and choose your words to set the course you desire. Like phrases used for hypnosis, design your subliminal message for success.

❁ Try This: The Body Channel

Once you've handled the habitual and emotional resistance, convincing your body to exercise isn't the tricky part. By now, it has gone through several cycles of being in and out of health and fitness. When you're out of shape your body feels dull, fatigued, and unhappy, with headaches, muscle and joint pains, grouchiness, cravings, and restlessness. When you're in shape, it's like riding a wave of good feeling, good energy, good inspiration, and good self-esteem. Like a pet, your body is eager to exercise. Delete the bad habits and negative thoughts, and you'll discover that your body wants and needs to move. When you turn on the Body Channel, the pleasure principle rules—it feels good to be limber, strong, and able to move with ease. Pain makes you feel crummy, stiff, weak, and unmotivated. The simple truths of anatomy and physiology are great motivators.

To make sure your fitness program is sustainable and enjoyable, make it body-centered. Whether you're in the gym, playing tennis, or walking to work, keep your focus on your body. Pay attention to moving parts, focused effort, and your beautiful mechanic design rather than trying to look good, do more, or be more. Keep your mind on what you're doing rather than chewing an emotional issue or working out a problem. Following are some tips for body-centered fitness:

- Check in with your body before you start.

- Get grounded and feel your feet on the earth, your pelvis on the seat.

- Stay loose and keep the motion fluid and easy.

- Let go of excess tension and avoid overexertion.

- Be aware of good posture and body mechanics.

- Stay focused on your body, keep your mind empty.

- Be grateful for your wise body.

As you practice body-centered fitness, it's natural to feel the tug of your dominating mind. But what if your mind took the hike with you instead of wandering off in another direction? Staying tuned in to your Body Channel can be a new and challenging experience when you usually:

- Read or listen to news on an exercise bike

- Talk to a friend while power walking

- Resolve emotional issues while you run

- Look for creative solutions in the lap lane

When you do body-centered exercise, it often tells you something about your mind. It will also give you new insights into the mechanics, feelings, changes, and challenges of your body. Remember, basic fitness isn't just about getting fit, it's also a way to get healthy. Practicing body-centered fitness helps you tune in and stay tuned. Like a moving meditation, it's a way to clear the holding patterns in your thoughts, emotions, and physical body. Regardless of your fitness level, your wise body has something to help you improve.

Rest and Sleep

Rest just doesn't happen on vacation or at the end of the day in your armchair. It's an essential part of your twenty-four-hour activity cycle. If you were to make a graph, you'd see a series of waves that flow from activity to rest, activity to rest, all day long. Taking a rest fits in nicely between telephone calls or on the walk to the restroom. It's any time when you take a breather to renew your energy and sharpen your focus. Dancers, athletes, and people who work with their body know the importance of resting and pacing themselves. But if your work is more mental than physical, you may forget your body's basic need to recharge. Let's face it: the cultural norm is to fuel the day with caffeine and adrenaline. Even a coffee (or lunch) break is hardly a break at all. It's surprising how difficult it is to factor in the body and do something so very natural. Did you ever think someone would have to tell you to practice taking it easy?

Your body functions best when its energy gets replenished. Like a work of art that has no negative space, your life simply has no definition without rest. Not only do you need rest physiologically, you need it for graceful living. Following are some opportunities to fit in a few moments of basic rest:

- At beginnings and endings (appointments, tasks, events)

- Between one task and the next

- Whenever you stop (at a traffic light, standing in line, in the waiting room)

- When it's your turn to listen in a conversation

- When you sit down to eat/lie down to sleep

During these rest periods, take a breather—literally *take three breaths in a row*. Just like your muscles need a rest cycle in order to function, so do you. When you come up against the resistance and persistence of your go-go-go habit, remind yourself that you're practicing something new and natural. Learning to exit the busy highway of life and pull into a rest stop will fill up your tanks so you don't have to tap your reserves. Just a few minutes of intentional rest pays off in steady energy resources all day long. If you want to live life fully and deeply rather than skim along the surface, master the art of rest.

Gary. *Over the years, Gary had spent hours and hours in the dentist's chair. How-ever, no matter how many visualization techniques he tried, he left the office feeling spent and exhausted. Determined to use his aware body to overcome the anxiety, Gary decided to dedicate his next appointment to practicing the art of rest. Instead of distracting himself and reading a magazine in the waiting room, he closed his eyes, tuned into his body, and let go of a layer of nervous tension. Once he was in the chair, his breath and the pull of gravity gently coaxed his muscles into rest even more. From this place, he could direct his positive visualization through rather than around his body—and he succeeded! With his hands resting on his belly, it was easy to feel comfort and reassurance with each movement of breath. As the dentist did his work, Gary used his time to rest a bit.*

As Gary discovered, letting go and resting is a good way to squelch fear and anxiety. Tending to basic rest is an everyday thing…and it can even happen at dental appointments! Factoring in rest is one of the basics for being alive. It's also one of the tools for survival. In the next chapter, you'll learn how to use your basic resting skills to handle stress.

The ultimate rest is sleep. Any twenty-four-hour cycle should have a big chunk set aside for sleep—eight to ten hours. Your body needs sleep in order to repair and replenish. Your mind needs sleep in order to sort and store emotional and mental input. This is how your body was designed. Without the benefit of deep rest, you get stressed physically/psychologically, and your mental functions become compromised. Even though you know it's good for you, getting good sleep might be a challenge, a variable, or an elusive experience. How can you drop down and turn it all off when your senses are overstimulated and your mind is constantly buzzing? Taking rest stops during the day will help you when the lights go out. When you're ready to go to sleep, everything you've learned about pausing and letting go gets put to good use. Like Gary discovered in the dentist's office, your body is not only the container for your tension and worries but also is the key for relaxation and rest. Meditation techniques focus on your breath and your senses simply because tuning in to your body helps you tune out your mind.

Even for people who have no problem, the process of falling asleep and staying asleep can be tricky. For people with sleep problems, it presents hurdles that seem insurmountable. Paying attention to your body can be a viable way to parlay simple resting into a good night's sleep. What you've learned in this book so far will help you address sleep in a body-centered way. For instance, you've learned about the shape of tension, habits of overachievement, and hypnotic self-talk. You've learned about the anatomy and physics of a moving, breathing body. You've practiced how to release excess tension and stay resilient in all your activities. You've tuned in to your personal needs and learned to trust your body a little more. You've challenged yourself to pause and rest during the day. Now take what you've learned to bed.

Knowing how to relax is a key to sleeping well. But how we actually transit from wakefulness to sleep remains a mystery. It turns out that the image of pixie dust isn't that far off! Even if you're dead tired, exhausted, and fall asleep the minute your head hits the pillow, how it happened continues to elude scientists. One thing we know is that going to sleep is not an active endeavor as much as it is a passive surrender. As any insomniac knows, you don't pursue sleep with any success—sleep simply finds you.

Find Your Sleep Zone

How can you set the scene so sleep can find you? Getting into the sleep zone starts at least a half hour before bedtime. This is your time to unwind from the day and prepare for the night. What is your typical routine? Do you cease stimulating activities and dim the lights to simulate dusk? Once in bed, it's time to settle in and quiet the mind chatter. This is not the time for mental figuring and emotional processing. Whether or not sleep comes easily, here are some ways to get in the zone where sleep can find you:

- Make sure your bedroom is comfortable, quiet, darkened, and uncluttered.

- Give yourself plenty of fresh, cool air.

- Set yourself up with a good mattress, ample pillows, and cozy covers.

- No TV, movies, provocative conversations, or intense and focused reading.

- Establish a set routine of self-care and sleep hygiene.

- Set up rituals like meditation or unchallenging, restorative yoga poses, or listening to peaceful music.

- Seek out and relax the muscular tensions of the day.

- Focus your mind on your breath—inhale to exhale to inhale to exhale.

Make a commitment to add a couple of these suggestions over the next few nights and notice if your quality of restful sleep improves. Was it easier for sleep to find you? Did your body help you quiet your mind? Was your sleep more fulfilling? Setting up good sleep conditions gets your body and mind in the sleep zone.

> *Jamie. When Jamie explored her bedtime routine, she realized that watching TV before sleep was counterproductive. For years she assumed that she was relaxing each night with the 10:00 pm news. After all, she was in her bed and dog-tired from her busy day. When she turned off the lights, however, she was anything but relaxed. It seemed to take forever to quiet her mind and surrender to a deeper layer of fatigue. It was as if her daytime self was fighting tooth and nail to stay in control. When she followed the sleep zone suggestions, she discovered that listening to music in her dimly lit bedroom was the perfect segue to sleepy time. When Jamie turned off the lights, she was already halfway there.*

Like Jamie, as you close out your day, it's important to empty your mind of its busyness (business) and quiet your body. Stimulating activities, solving emotional problems, or answering emails right up to the threshold of sleep doesn't allow your system to decompress. Without an interlude between activity and sleep, some of the intensity of your overly stimulated life carries on right into your sleep. Bedtime is your time to tune in, soften tension, and be quietly at home in your body. This is as important as brushing your teeth and washing your face.

❁ Try This: A Good Night's Sleep

When you include body wisdom, you can change your mind about sleeping. Use the following imagery to help you get a good night's sleep: Like a boat drifting into the current, it's just you and your body casting off and floating along to sleep. To let go of the shore and let yourself be carried away, check in with your body and let each microspace of tension soften and seep away. With each exhale, send your random thoughts away like so many particles into the sky. With each inhale, fill yourself with soft acceptance of all that is. Let your sense of space expand around your body and beyond—this is the sleep zone; linger here. Keep feeling how your body undulates softly with each breath and your mind expands into soft spaciousness. This is your sleep zone, where the deep rest of sleep can find you. What if your body was held in the soothing comfort of "spirit" while your mind drifted away to sleep?

> *Violet. As long as she could remember, Violet's body felt wired and antsy. It was hard for her to quiet down and rest anytime, day or night. The savasana pose for winding down at the end of a yoga class was anything but restful! She didn't know what she was expected or supposed to do and felt like a failure. Her overactive mind and muscles also made it hard to get to sleep and stay asleep. Fashioning her own "sleep yoga," Violet cleverly combined a resting pose with images from a popular children's book. Lying in bed before sleep, she relaxed her body to the cadences of the children's book,* Goodnight Moon. *Saying "goodnight neck, goodnight nose, goodnight feet with little toes," she visited each place in her body with loving regard. As she put her body to sleep, her mind was put to rest as well. Just like a child, her dear body rested easier when it felt soothed and tucked in for the night.*

Aesthetics

Taking care of the aesthetics in your life may not seem basic to your well-being, but it is—you need space, design, beauty, and love. Poets and philosophers throughout the ages have extolled the importance of such aesthetics for your mind and soul but they're also imperative for your body. Through biochemistry and brain imaging research, scientists have linked the vibrancy of your body to basic aesthetics.[2] Tending to the art of living is simply essential to your body's health and happiness. Below are some ways to accomplish the art of living.

....

2   Anjan Chatterjee, "The Aesthetic Brain," in *Oxford Scholarship Online,* accessed Jan 2014. www.oxfordscholarship.com/view/10.1093/acprof:oso/9780199811809.001.0001 /acprof-9780199811809.

Ample Space

The space you need is as personal as your own body. When you have enough space, you feel comfortable and move with ease. When you don't, it creates stress and tension. For example, if your clothes are too tight, your body feels restricted; if you're crowded by clutter, your body feels claustrophobic. Your body also has an individualized sense of social space and intimacy. Some people handle the condensed space of crowds easily; others don't. Some people sleep better spooning, others can't even share a room. Listen to your body, it'll tell you if it has ample space. To figure out how much space you need, let your body be your measuring stick. Anytime it feels compressed, crowded, or tense, your body may need more space. Sometimes more space means wide, open spaces. Did you ever notice that spending time in nature—city parks, a path in the woods, a mountain meadow, or even your own backyard—seems to replenish and renew your energy?

> *Carol. As a dermatologist, Carol needed space to move around her patients and access various products and equipment. Working in a treatment room that was too small, she soon discovered the importance of basic space. Because she was constantly reaching, scrunching, and twisting, her body took on the restrictions of her workstation. The "crowded" feeling in her hips and lower back became a chronic problem that brought her to a surgeon's door. To truly repair the damage, Carol needed to make the connection between her cramped workstation and her body pains. When she rearranged things so her body could move freely and did some physical therapy, her back began to heal. With the space she needed, not only could her body move but her work flowed as well.*

Good Design

The ergonomics of anything you use—your desk, car, kitchen, tools, and so on—need to support your body no matter what you're doing. Bodies come in different sizes and shapes, so one size will *not* fit all. The height of your desk, the firmness of your bed, the tilt of your car's seat, the shape of your backpack, and the weight of your tennis racket should all fit you as surely as your shoes. If these particulars are designed well, your body can move easily, work efficiently, and avoid undue stress or injury. A simple rule of thumb is to ensure your environment is accommodating you, not the other way around.

Paul. Because Paul's desk was too low, his body invariably ended up slumping. Not only did this poor posture create muscle tension, it also restricted his breathing, eyesight, ability to move, and his mood. To feel better at work, Paul needed to consider the design variables of his own body. With his desk higher, he could move and breathe easier and had more energy at the end of the day. With his head higher, his eyes were less strained and his outlook improved. Out of the slump, Paul could see the possibility of solutions. When he looked "on top of it" rather than downtrodden, people responded to him differently. Good design helped Paul's body and his career.

Sensual Beauty

From the very beginning of your life, your eyes have been drawn to symmetry and color. A baby prefers the face of its mother and tracks certain colors and forms with fascination. Experiments have shown how appealing visuals can trigger "feel-good" hormones and become associated with sensual pleasure. Look around as you go about your day and give yourself a perk. Here are some examples of beauty that might delight your eyes:

- The delightful contrast of color in a work of art

- The athletic grace of a dog jumping for a ball

- The symmetry in the face of a loved one

- The dance of storm clouds racing across the sky

- The symphony of birds singing at dawn

Whenever you see, smell, feel, hear, or even imagine beauty, your body's physiology registers pleasure. This reinforces your basic sense of aesthetics. You're drawn to the smell of a rose, the touch of velvet, the sound of a babbling brook, the movement of dance, or the play of dappled sunlight on a wall. You relax just a bit. Have you ever noticed your body expand, sigh, and feel a sense of well-being when your eye landed on something beautiful?

Sue. Sue told me how she'd transformed a dismal, unattractive flat she had in London when she was younger and poorer. Tending to her basic need for aesthetics, Sue placed her belongings just so—a colorful cloth here and an arrangement of beach glass there. When her landlady came for a visit, she commented, "Nothing really has changed here but something you have done makes it look so much better!" Sue had just added her sense of beauty. Not only did the flat look better but it felt better as well. No matter how stringent the budget, including basic beauty is good for your body.

A Bit of Love

Just like a plant or a pet, your body responds favorably to love and appreciation. You know the phrase "failure to thrive"? With a constant diet of neglect and criticism, it makes sense that your body ends up looking and feeling haggard. Eventually, the message takes a toll on your well-being. As with any primary relationship, your body needs to know that you care. Your body isn't picky, anything caring counts. Listed below are some suggestions:

- Anytime you think of it, tell your body how grateful you are for its strength, health, limberness, and faithfulness.

- Check in with your body and its comfort. Make sure your posture/ position has the support it needs.

- Respond when your body gives you the pain/pressure/distress signal. This is telling you to do something! Get up, go for a walk, change the ergonomics, buy new shoes, see a professional for help, and take action.

- Pay attention to the fine tuning. Do you have the energy, digestion (elimination), libido, and sleep you need? Take the necessary steps to correct any imbalances through diet or exercise or rest.

- Treat yourself as you would a beloved. Regard your basic care/regular maintenance as an act of love and, now and then, give yourself little gifts and vacations.

There are many ways to give your body the love it needs. Depending on your personality, your expression of self-love might be a new sweat suit, dinner out, or a day at the beach. Like any other living thing, *your body needs love in order to thrive*. Taking care of your basic needs from breathing and eating consciously to giving yourself the rest, exercise, support, and beauty you need is a powerful way to say "I love you" to your body. This is the kind of love that goes a long way and lasts a lifetime.

Tending to your basic needs sets the groundwork for the rest of your life. Establish good self-care practices and your body gets the message. When you stop taking your body for granted and start including it as an important part of the program, you set something very powerful in motion. When it's not stressed or silenced, your body continues to wake up, share wisdom, and claim its rightful place next to your mind and spirit. Understanding the intelligence and importance of your body changes your perspective on everything. Now that you have the basics in place, you have the foundation to explore some crucial and timely topics, such as stress and relaxation, injury and illness, emotional intelligence, intimacy and intuition, spirit, and the quality of life.

Four
Stress and Relaxation

Understanding the importance of living fully and carefully in your body changes your relationship with your body. You no longer take it for granted—you don't ignore, boss, or bully. Your new partnership is helping you pay attention in new ways. As you tuned in and tended to the basics of self-care, you may have been surprised to find pockets of tension and stress tucked here and there in your body. Chronic tension can seem normal and fly under the radar of everyday awareness; after so much time, it simply feels like who you are. Honestly though, do you really need to squeeze your forehead in order to read or brace your shoulders in order to drive? Does pushing your tongue against your teeth help you balance the checkbook? Does tightening your buttocks make chopping vegetables easier? Some excess stress-load is physical and rooted in poor posture and movement habits, while some is emotional and sourced in unresolved feelings and attitudinal habits. But as any health care professional will tell you, these chronic tension habits aren't benign—they can have a profound and negative effect on your health, happiness, and vitality, now and in the future. It's time to let your wise body teach you how to release and relax.

In the past ten years, brain imaging technology and cell physiology research have established an irrefutable connection between mind and body. Today, science can confirm what your personal experience has known for a long time: that chronic physical tension isn't good for your state of mind and chronic mental stress isn't good for your physical health and performance.[3] You don't need to understand the intricacies of the research in order to benefit from the findings. You personally verify the efficacy of the mind-body relationship anytime you answer the questions: Where am I storing my stress? What is the source of this stress-load? How can I decrease stress factors in my life? And, how can I improve my relaxation skills?

You know what stress feels like. Simply being alive today means you've experienced personal challenges, creative conundrums, workload deadlines, unexpected changes, financial uncertainty, emotional disappointment, and times of global and environmental crisis. You've felt the surge of adrenaline when a fellow driver cuts you off. You've felt your stomach clutch during a difficult telephone call. You've felt the unrelenting tension in your neck when your schedule lacks downtime. These feelings of surge, clutch, and tension are natural responses to specific situations. If tension carries over from one situation to the next, however, being tense may soon become the norm. Your body can forget how to relax due to performance demands, tight schedules, and information overload. Stress piles on top of stress and your nervous system scrambles to accommodate an unrelenting, low-grade, perpetual hyperarousal. Like working muscles, your nervous system needs recovery time in order to perform well and stay healthy. If left unattended, stress will build up until it reaches a tipping point and your health and performance will plummet.

Sharon. Sharon was a high achiever and managed her stress by just trying harder. While flying home from a visit to family a couple of years ago, she felt anxious and couldn't catch her breath. Over the next few days, even with prescribed antianxiety medication she still felt jumpy 24/7. Sharon had hit the wall and her adrenals were shot. In order to regain health, her doctor told her to cut out anything stressful in her life—including caffeine and her exercise regimen—and learn to meditate. You see, Sharon had gotten used to living in a state of increased sensory stimulation and thought it was normal. Her stressfulness, however, was unsustainable. She realized that all her success would get her nowhere if she lost her health. It was time to learn about stress and relaxation.

....

3   Mayo Clinic Staff, "Stress Symptoms: Effects on Your Body and Behavior," Mayo Clinic, accessed May 2017. www.mayoclinic.org/healthy-lifestyle/stress-management/in-depth /stress-symptoms/art-20050987.html.

Before you sustain a health crisis, it may be prudent to take a look at the causes and effects of stress in your life. No matter how facile you are, carrying extra stress doesn't make sense when you don't have to. To assess if your own health might be compromised by stressful life habits, answer the following questions:

- Do you have difficulty falling asleep at night?

- Is it easy for you to sit quietly and do nothing?

- When you're doing something routine, do you double up and multitask?

- When plans change, do you scramble to fill your calendar?

- Do you alternate work/play/rest activities throughout your day?

- Do you allow the space for a full breath no matter what you are doing?

- Do you perceive yourself as a *human being* or a *human doing*?

The truth is, your system is hardwired to respond to life-threatening events. This is good for you and can even save your life. However, it's bad for you when fight-or-flight physiology triggers over and over in response to random loud noises, congested traffic, emotional upset, work demands, or unexpected change. Learning to manage the mundane, everyday stress in your world is truly the health challenge of the twenty-first century, and your wise body is here to help. Here's a three-step process to turn it all around: (1) find the stress, (2) develop body-oriented strategies to let it go, (3) practice body-centered relaxation every day.

Stress

Stress is carried in your tight muscles. You might be surprised to discover how much unnecessary tension accompanies even simple activities like brushing your teeth or holding a coffee cup. Even on the most relaxing vacation, you might be carrying some extra baggage in your tense shoulders and, after a long, restful sleep you may still be clenching your jaw. Bring your awareness to your body anytime of day or night and you'll find at least one area in your body overtight and overworking. Chances are the particular pattern of tension you find isn't so random. It's your particular way of holding on and your own unique *shape of stress*. Carrying this extra tension is unhealthy and not the way your body works best.

The Shape of Stress

How does your body work best? At a physiological level, your body works best when it knows the difference between the tiger and the butterfly. If you sense the tiger, your body runs; if it's the butterfly, your body relaxes. At a purely physical level, your body works best when effort matches the activity. For heavy work, you need more muscle; for light work, you need less. Any muscular tension beyond the task simply gets in the way. For instance, when you're driving, conditions will determine how you hold the steering wheel. Some conditions call for a directive, light touch; others may require a firmer grasp for rapid response. Many people don't differentiate and hold the wheel tightly no matter what, as if driving conditions were hazardous and life depended on it. If you want to be safe and drive well, habitually gripping the wheel is counterproductive. It adds unnecessary stress, and your braced muscles make your response time slower and your coordination clumsier.

❋ *Try This: Stressful Tension*

Your muscles are working right now as you read this book: postural muscles make sure you don't slump; jaw muscles keep your mouth closed; hand and arm muscles hold the book; and eye muscles track the words. Your muscles might be overworking even with an activity that's hardly physical. Let's check it out: Pause for a moment and let your hands rest, your eyes soften, and your jaw/face relax. Now, pay attention to what happens to your eyes as you squeeze your hands/arms. Flex and let go a few times. Did your eyes seem to tighten and let go as well? This kind of secondary tension has nothing to do with reading and actually hinders your eyes' ability to focus and track. Maybe you don't want to be gripping the book as if it's going to get away from you.

Anytime you have excessive tension in one part of your body, your whole body tenses up just a little (squeeze your calves and see if your neck tightens a bit). Overmuscling everything, from the steering wheel to the dog leash to the book in hand, creates and sustains your personal shape of stress. Paying attention to where and when you overmuscle helps you identify chronic holding patterns, reduces overall stress, and allows you to enjoy life a bit more. Anything you do can be more relaxing if you don't overmuscle. When you swing a hammer, you'll need the help of your arm, shoulder, and stomach muscles, not your jaw. When you brush your teeth, the lightest touch gets the job done. And like hitting the refresh button on your computer, after you've finished an activity, make sure you let go of the workload and pause for a moment.

Observe your body in any activity and you may be surprised to find excess muscle tension. You're overworking if your jaw tightens when you carry a heavy load. You're overworking if your forehead scrunches when shampooing your hair. You're overworking if your stomach carries nervous tension. You're overworking if your fists clench when you're running.

> *George.* *George felt the shape of stress after a last-minute dash to catch the subway. Even after he'd found a seat, his jaw was clamped and he held his newspaper as if it was going to blow away. When he let go of this excess tension, he was able to take a few moments of respite before his busy day began.*

> *Lila.* *Lila was amused to find some ridiculous tension when she was walking her dog on the beach one day. As usual, her dog was eager to get out and sniff around and, naturally, Lila needed a firm grip on the leash in her right hand. However, her left hand was also gripping with equal intensity. When she let go of this extra work, she began to enjoy some playfulness of her own.*

> *Bianca.* *After her last exam, Bianca felt like she could finally relax, but she found herself bolting up from bed and powering around her dorm room as if it was still finals week. She needed to let go of the shape of stress before it was possible to slow down and take some well-deserved time off. As was said in the old Psalm: "there's a time to work and a time to rest."*

The key to finding the stress is to pay attention to your body. Is your muscle tension calibrated for what you're doing right now? Are old habits and tension patterns the reason for the pain in your tight stomach, jaw, or calves? Is it hard to let go and let your body function in its optimal design? Do you carry your shape of stress into sleep?

If you hold the impression of an uptight lifestyle everywhere you go, you'll never have the space to relax and enjoy the moment. When you and your muscles don't know how to relax, tension self-perpetuates and stress accumulates.

✿ Try This: The Stress-o-Meter

Imagine a scale that measures action/relaxation for any given activity. Each thing you do registers the select muscles and tensile strength necessary to accomplish the task at hand. At one extreme, resting and sleeping require no muscle work and major relaxation. Because you don't need your shoulders scrunched or your forehead furled, this tension would increase your score on the stress-o-meter. For lifting, driving, or typing, you need a specific amount of tension to do the job. If you overmuscle, your score goes up on the stress-o-meter. Pay attention over the next few days to your body tension and see how you score. The following *in-between* times can shine a spotlight on your action/relaxation ratio:

- When you wake up in the morning, do you feel rested and begin your day slowly? Or, does your body feel pumped with the tension of an emotional issue, looming deadline, or simple habit?

- When you walk to your car do your arms and legs swing easily? Do you feel a bouncy reverb with each step? Do your eyes notice the world around you? Or, are your hands jammed in your pockets, your feet pounding the pavement, and/or your eyes fixed on the ground?

- When you break for lunch, do you truly take a break and show up for eating, relaxing, and socializing? Or, do you take your work out to lunch and forget to enjoy the food and company?

- After you put away groceries, do you take a moment to breathe and let go of the effort of shopping and schlepping? Or, does your body stay cocked for action as you power on to check your emails and fix dinner?

- When you settle in after dinner to read or watch TV, do you set yourself up for comfort? Can you feel your back relax into the sofa and your breath move easily in your belly? Or, do you perpetuate the tension of the day in all your favorite places? Do you push beyond fatigue to accomplish more work and end up too wired to settle down?

These in-between moments of transitioning from one part of your day to another are great times to wake up and listen to your wise body. When you find places that are over-muscling, see if you can let them go. Checking your stress-o-meter throughout the day pinpoints the particulars of your *shape of stress* and highlights the changes you need to make. This doesn't take extra time; it takes awareness and intention. Letting go of over-muscling not only helps you de-stress, it keeps tension from becoming hypertension. It's simple math.

What Is the Math?

You can think of stress as a function of addition and subtraction. Increasing or decreasing tension is a math that begins in the morning and continues all day long. You're not starting off at zero if you wake up and your jaw is clenched so much your teeth hurt, your shoulders are up around your ears, and your belly is so tight it is hard to breathe. First thing, you'll need to do some subtraction so you don't add on stress to stress. How you start your day sets the baseline.

It's important to get a fresh start each day. You wouldn't wear yesterday's dirty clothes, so why wear yesterday's stress? In order to get a fresh start, come to your senses and begin your day with zero stress. Here's how: When you awaken, take a moment to hear the birds (murmur of traffic or wind in the trees) and let your eyes survey the soft morning light. You don't have to bolt out of bed—take all the time you need in the next few minutes, there's no rush. Start moving your body slowly as you gently shake the sleepy tension out of your arms/legs and roll easily out of bed. Stand up and let your spine/neck and hips shift and rotate to get the circulation going and release any stiffness. Feel the lift of your head toward the sky and the support of the ground under your feet. As you inhale, feel your readiness for the fresh day ahead and step into it. The break of day is a great time to begin anew. Remember, don't let yesterday's stress burden today's possibilities.

Subtracting tension at the beginning (and throughout) your day will reduce the sum of stress in your body. Anytime you can let go of stress, you make room for more focus and vitality. When you get to the end of the day, it just makes sense to do a major tension dump.

The end of the day is a good time to subtract some stress tension. Focus on your body in the interlude between work and not-work and use your anatomical breathing to dislodge any residual worries and concerns. Let all of the stuck, hard, tight places give way to the gentle motion of your breath. Let the impressions, challenges, and intensity of the day float away with each exhale. Taking the stress of your workday into your time off is simply counterproductive. When you end with a sum of stress, you'll need to do some subtraction so it doesn't accompany you on into the night.

As you practice, you'll get better and better at reducing your stress numbers and letting tension dissipate. It will be second nature to check in, notice the extra tension, and let it go. Over time you'll become adept at dissembling your shape of stress whenever it happens. A few moments before an important meeting, after a challenging event, or during in-between times can make a huge difference between whether you're overtaxed, stressed out, and spun out—or calm, confident, and relaxed. As you continue to practice, your body-mind will get a new message and layers of overmuscling habits will simply dissolve.

History of Stress

Once you find stress in your body, you may wonder how it got there in the first place. Beyond simple functional habits and lack of awareness, your *shape of stress* may have its own story. To address the source, you may need to look at some personal and emotional history. Ever since you were born, you've been sculpting the shape of your own personal stress. This process is generally unconscious, ongoing, and cumulative. Each time you faced a challenge, difficulty, or the unknown, your body responded. Each time you encountered fear, frustration, or confusion, your emotions responded. In their unique way, these physical and emotional moments have shaped who you are. Key experiences in your personal history can become hardwired in your posture and tension patterns. Once you find the stress and address the source, you're in a position to address the unconscious habitual tension and leave history behind. What if each time you encountered a tricky situation, you used your body wisdom to diffuse tension rather than take it on?

✾ *Try This: Your Stress Footprint*

What's the emotional history of your tension patterns? A great time to identify how stress translates to tension is when you're tired and spent at the end of a hard day. Check in with your body and feel where you're heavy, braced, or restricted. Notice the quality of expression in this shape of stress when you squeeze, slump, or furrow a little more. What emotions and attitudes does this shape embody? What story does it tell you? When fear lives in the shape of your collapsed chest, your body will return to it every time you're uncertain or scared. When anger lives in your clenched fists, your hands will tighten every time you feel slighted or ignored. When sadness lives in your slumped shoulders, it's hard to find joy and exuberance. As I often say, your history determines your shape, and eventually, your shape determines your history. Instead of holding on, let it go right now: shrug your shoulders, wiggle your jaw, move your brow up and down, expand your chest. Whatever it takes to get it moving! Move it on and imagine the emotional story is shaking loose and moving on as well. It's true that the body holds your history, but it can also let it go.

In the natural course of progressive bodywork and somatic therapy, my clients often run into their personal history. Ed's sagging shoulders carried an anger that started way back in elementary school where he'd often felt inadequate. When he let go of the shape of this story, his body no longer felt like it wanted to curl up and hide whenever he faced difficulty at the office. Joe's jutting jaw and hunched shoulders held an anger that could be traced to his older sister's bullying. When he let go of the shape of this story, his body could stand in its power without having to feel like a bulldog holding its ground. And, Nan's pinching eyebrows held the confusion of a little girl looking for approval. When she let go of the shape of this story, she could recognize her accomplishments and give herself the appreciation she needed. Feeling the influence of the past in their present-day bodies gave all of these clients something to focus on to change the future. Shaking, softening, expanding, and letting go is a good way to dislodge your emotional shape of stress. When you're not carrying yesterday's hurt, confusion, disgust, uncertainty, and so forth you can make a good impression today. Diminishing the emotional component of your stress footprint frees you up to be aware, confident, focused, and relaxed.

Undoing your shape of stress is like letting go of a bad habit—it takes a little time and a lot of awareness. Drop in now and then to see if there's some place in your body that's holding on ... *you* know where to look.

Strategies for Letting Go

Stress happens. You've explored how, where, and why you carry a shape of stress. How can you minimize and manage stress when it inevitably happens? Here are seven powerful strategies to help you navigate in a stressful world: become aware, change your mindset, don't multitask, slow down, limit exposure, and enjoy life.

Become Aware

Becoming more aware will help you let go. You've been practicing and now it's time to use your body awareness to monitor tension, bracing, and over-muscling. Use your body sense to deliver just the right amount of muscle effort to daily activities like walking the dog, brushing your hair, carrying your suitcase, playing the piano, etc. Break the tension habit of accumulating stress from morning to night, activity to activity. Notice if the effort of scrubbing a pot walks with you across the room to turn off the light. Notice if the left bicep is tight while the right arm brushes your hair. If you're always adding rather than subtracting tension, relaxation will be an elusive concept. Develop a routine of letting go of your shape of stress first thing in the morning and in between activities all day long. You'll need to practice this body mindfulness maybe for the rest of your life in order to become aware and change the ingrained, unconscious habits of overtensing muscles.

> *Gregory.* *Gregory felt some jitters before giving a public speech. On his walk to the lecture hall, he shook his upper body and freed up a bit of anxiety. Letting his body move easily also helped, yet something was still holding on. Scanning his body, he found the culprit in the overmuscling of his hand carrying his briefcase. It felt as if some energy was blocked and tension went up his arm and shoulder. When he softened his grip, his arms could swing with ease and the tension dissipated. Those few minutes of self-awareness helped Gregory walk up to the podium with his expertise and charm. Being aware and letting go beforehand meant that his stress wasn't part of his presentation.*

Being body aware is a good way to "work smarter, not harder." Working smarter means approaching anything you do like a dance. No matter how mundane, focusing on balance and grace will help you find ease and fun. Even when leaning over to pick up a pencil, let your whole body move fluidly. It's an illusion that the fewer body parts you use, the more efficient and less stressful work is. Your body's parts are mechanically designed to move cooperatively whether you're loading lumber or conducting an orchestra. You create excess tension and put your body on hold whenever you use one part and immobilize the rest. Letting your body move fully in its mechanical design, invigorates your energy and diminishes stress.

> *Kate.* *Kate was helping her partner stack firewood for the winter. As she went along, the logs felt heavier and heavier. This hard work was straining her back and arms. She realized that she was holding back from the task, not using her whole body and paying attention to the ramblings of her mind. When she remembered to unlock her hips and use her whole body in this menial task, it became more like a game of "stack the wood." Her body felt less tense and the logs seemed lighter. When the woodpile was finished, her energy felt replenished, rather than depleted. Being outdoors and moving her body helped her take a break from her problems and de-stress.*

Change Your Mindset

See stressful times as opportunities. No one gets through life stress-free. As a matter of fact, there's substantial argument that stress actually helps you learn, mature, and grow. It's like the pearl in the oyster; it won't grow without a little irritation. But, you want to harvest your pearls without taking on an attitude of aggravation, blame, and defeat. Acknowledging and accepting stress as a natural part of life means keeping your cool when things fall apart. It means taking care of your body as a valuable partner and resource. Instead of being stoic or a superhero, ask for help. Instead of loading on extra work, social commitments, or junk food to distract your feelings, give your body a break. Gauge your relaxation needs and tell your inner worker bee that it's okay to slack off a bit. Rather than deplete you resources, why not replenish them? Nurture your body with a massage, facial, pedicure, or a few hours at a spa. Create some time to listen to music or a guided meditation CD, eat dinner with friends, sit in the winter sun, or take a vacation to help you through stressful times.

Donald. Donald's mother had been ill for some time and he thought he was pre- pared for her eventual demise. But when she finally passed, the extra stress buried him. His normal pattern was to go into high gear, handle the situation, and not ask for help. As his mental distraction became apparent, his boss urged him to take some time off for R and R. Instead of powering on, Donald needed to pause and acknowl- edge this landmark moment in his life. When he checked in with himself, his body seemed so sidelined with exhaustion that his mind felt unmoored and rudderless. The old way of filling his calendar with activity and his stomach with "comfort food" made things worse rather than better. So Donald did something really unusual—he changed his attitude. Instead of overriding his feelings and powering through, he cleared his calendar, joined a bereavement support group, and gave himself the tenderness he needed to heal. When Donald emerged at the other end of his grief, he took his learning with him. No longer was stress a random inconvenience; it was a wake-up call to pay attention and take care of himself.

Don't Multitask

Multitasking is stressful. You may be proud of your ability to multitask, but it's not good for your health. Science is now discovering that multitasking isn't multitracking. Rather than do two or more things at once, your brain shifts its focus back and forth, back and forth. It turns out that focusing on more than one thing at once is not only inefficient but it also affects your clarity, accuracy, and stress levels.[4] Every injured carpenter will tell you that they were thinking of something else when the accident happened. But multitasking habits can be very hard to break. Simply observe your routines for a short while and see how prevalent multitasking is in your life. Following are some ways you might be doubling up:

- Listening to voice mail while brushing your teeth or walking to the car

- Sending text messages at a concert, lecture, or restaurant

- Talking to someone while checking email

....

4   Issie Lapowsky, "Don't Multitask: Your brain will thank you," in *Time*, April 17, 2013 business.time.com/2013/04/17/dont-multitask-your-brain-will-thank-you/.html.

- Driving while eating, putting on makeup, or talking on a cell phone
- Making a mental to-do list while reading aloud to a child or receiving a massage

It might surprise you to find how many variations of multitasking you can fit into an average day. A powerful way to subtract some stress from your day is to take the challenge to stop multitasking. Do only one thing at a time. Cultivate a compartmentalized approach to each activity and moment. When you walk in nature, only walk in nature. When you read, commit yourself to reading. When you listen to music, singularly enjoy the music. Finish one task before you begin or even think of the next.

Jemma. Jemma was starting her own business and her days were packed. Her life was consumed with work. When she was eating, exercising, walking her dogs, or getting a pedicure she was thinking about work. When she was social, sexual, or sleeping she was thinking about work. Rather than producing results, juggling all her balls at once was exhausting. When she stopped letting her work bleed through to every corner of her life, Jemma got the true rest she needed when she slept, the true love she needed when she was out with friends, the true play she needed when she was at the gym, and the true nourishment she needed when she sat down to eat. Instead of compounding stress, learning to "single task" gave Jemma the focus she needed to make the decisions, see the potential, tap the creativity, and pitch the product of her new business.

Slow Down

It's hard to slow down. Going at high speed is understandable when you live in a demanding and distracting world. But, as anyone with adrenal exhaustion can tell you, time can't be squeezed without a price to pay. This is how it works: as time compresses, your muscular and mental tension compress as well. You experience this when you're in a hurry and your body tightens up to do things faster. Did you know that tightening up just gets in your way? Think how impatient and jumpy people get when they're running late. The time it takes to accomplish a task is always influenced by physical constraints. If you go too fast, you upset the equation, make more mistakes, invite injury, and feel uptight. Slowing down is a good way to de-stress and relax. What if you actually drove the speed limit instead of five or ten miles over it? Truly, in this culture you'd need to get in the slow lane!

> *John Paul. John Paul prided himself in how fast he could accomplish a task. As a house painter, this was seen as a virtue and his hard work earned him a great reputation. But, because he was going so fast, he made mistakes that cost him time, money, and peace of mind. It seemed that all he did was work, and indeed it was making him a boring playmate. When he challenged himself to slow down and take a break now and then, he was baffled to discover that he got more done and felt less fatigue and stress at the end of the day. Now, he had time left over for leisure and play in his life. With his new schedule, he was renewed, ready, and eager for work the next day.*

Limit Exposure

Limit exposure to anything that stirs up stress. Most likely, the evening news is not your personal news. You want to know what's going on, but when you tune in to dramatic world events and inflammatory cultural dialogue, you turn on the "stress channel." Keeping abreast of the news doesn't mean putting it in your chest. Notice what happens to your body the next time the media hooks you with an unfolding catastrophe. Even if the story is about a weather system someplace far away, your body may follow along as if it was in your backyard. To limit exposure to the stress of world events, don't turn on the news every time you get in the car or come home from work. Listen to some music or the quiet passing of time. If you happen to get snagged into a stressful conversation or news segment, make sure to literally brush or shake it off your body afterward.

As a stress management strategy, it makes sense to limit exposure to some people you know and places you go. These can be tension generators and energy drains. How can you tell? Just pay attention to how your body feels. If you notice your mood deflated and feel tired after spending time with a friend, family member, or colleague, limit the time you spend with these people. If you have a headache or feel spent after being in crowded places, superstores, or rock concerts, listen to your body. Just putting your body in these situations can be overstimulating and needlessly stressful. Honor your own limits.

Josie. *Josie is an introvert. She's in her comfort zone when solving problems and being creative on her own. Even though her friends thought she was a good listener, Josie didn't know how to listen to her own body. Time and time again, she would accept invitations to big public events because she thought she needed to get out and get over her shyness. However, when her energy was inevitably zapped, she judged it as weakness or inadequacy when really her body was talking to her. When she stopped overriding and listened to her body, it was easy to make choices that limited her exposure to stress. For her, taking a hike in the wilderness was the best form of getting out. This was Josie's key to reduce the stress in her life.*

For some people, limiting exposure means changing or rearranging work, social, or family plans. For all people, taking a phone/texting/social media break every once in a while can be a stress-reducing strategy. Today, it's pretty easy to pack in so much content, there's no room left to just BE. For many people, limiting the constant exposure to external stimuli is necessary to even *feel* what's really going on. If you've grown accustomed to a sensory world that's loud, demanding, and pervasive you may need to limit your exposure in order to feel your body at all. You could be surprised at how much stress you've been carrying that's not yours at all.

Enjoy Life

Enjoying life is a delight to the senses. Eating, bathing, having sex, strolling in the park, holding a baby, and even exercising and physical labor can be delightful with the right mindset. If you take the time to enjoy a leisurely meal with friends, a breathtaking panoramic view, the fascinating repertoire of a mockingbird, the seductive scent of a rose, and the caress of a sweet breeze on a hot day, you're giving yourself *pleasure*. But, to truly partake of these pleasures, you may need to become more aware, change your attitude, lighten up, be present, slow down, and eliminate stressful distractions. There's an either-or relationship between pleasure and stress. After all, they just don't inhabit the same frame of mind, do they?

Your health care professional will tell you that stress is bad for your health. It's also bad for your state of mind and ability to be a creative, clear, loving, insightful, and even trustworthy person. Not only will stress hamper the quality of your life but, if left unattended, it can take you down. Managing stress with antianxiety medication, distraction, and denial only addresses symptoms. When you learn how to unravel habitual tension and develop personalized stress-reduction strategies, you can get underneath the symptoms. When you change the way you interact with the pace and circumstances of life, you can begin to change your shape of stress. Like so many of the examples earlier, when you pay attention to your wise body, it will show you what's holding on and how to let it go. What if your familiar state-of-body was relaxation instead of tension? What if you knew how to avoid stress in the first place? No matter what's happening in your life, it's time to practice some relaxation skills.

Learn to Relax

You need to learn how to relax in order to know how to relax. All your strategies to divert and manage stress and tension become much more effective when you become adept at relaxation. It's like coming at a problem from both sides. Simply sitting with your feet up at the end of the day is a good start though you may need to follow some advice and practice for years in order to master the art.

Relaxation

Relax Your Body

As you've discovered, your body is the vessel that carries your stress. However, your habits, mindset, and cultural milieu are at the control board. As you've gotten better at identifying and modifying your *shape of stress,* you've established new reference points for relaxation. Yet, for some people, true relaxation can still feel like an elusive goal. If your tension is rooted in emotional history and reinforced by years of accommodation, it may be hard to extract the *you* from the pattern. Even some highly physical people, such as athletes and dancers, can't translate the words *relax, let go,* or *loosen up* in their bodies.

> **Tom.** *Tom felt frustrated as he set out to find the source of his TMJ (chronic jaw tension) pain. No matter how hard he tried or how many massages he got, he just couldn't let it go. His jaw tension seemed as much a part of his identity as his black hair and brown eyes. He could even see the pervasive clench in his childhood photographs. When I asked him to relax his jaw, it meant nothing. As a young tennis star, he'd been under enormous pressure to focus and perform. His way of handling the*

tension was to store it in the set of his jaw. Presently, Tom is very facile in handling high-pressure situations, but his jaw still brings along the old message of striving and uncertainty. Although the circumstances have changed, his muscles still hold on to their old understanding. He needs to practice some body-focused relaxation in order to show up and be successful.

Learning how to relax your anatomy is the formula for unraveling tension any time, any place. The process is based on a simple concept: your body is composed of moving parts and when you tense up, your muscles clamp down and restrict the natural flow of movement. Nevertheless, you can reverse the process and let your body mechanics help you relax. Following is an exercise to help you circumvent the hold of the past and find a new reference point for relaxation:

- Find someplace in your body that feels tense. No matter where it is (neck, shoulders, butt, calves), shift your attention to the space underneath the tension and move your bones around a bit. Slowly, respectfully, move your bones—up, down, around, through, back, and forth. No matter where you find tension, get your anatomy moving and you'll dislodge it. Then, get your muscles moving—squeeze, jiggle, swing, and bounce. This is not about being athletic, this is about soft, juicy, and easy motion. Try the following:
  - Your jaw moves open and closed, side to side, forward and back
  - Your tongue moves around your teeth—front, back, and side to side
  - Your lips stretch, pout, push, and pucker
  - Your shoulders lift, rotate, shrug, slide, and shake
  - Your legs and hips roll, jiggle, sway, and swing

Just move your body slowly, gently, and intentionally to free up any logjam of tension and get things moving again. Without the tension, your body parts move freely and cooperatively in the way they were designed. If moving around and letting go brings up unsettling feelings, such as fear, anger, uncertainty, awkwardness, or sorrow, check out chapter 6 on emotional embodiment. If moving like this makes you feel playful and joyful, you've just relaxed a bit more. When you go through your body and let it help you relax, you demystify your tension. Each time you remind your overbusy, overstimulated body to keep it all moving, you undermine the hold of stress in your life. Your own moving body gives you a simple, personal way to unravel tension patterns and negotiate stress whenever it happens.

How did body-focused relaxation help our tennis player, Tom? Because the tension was so established in his jaw muscles, it was difficult to free up its natural movement. When he first moved his jaw side to side, movement was jerky and his chin quivered. When he tried to move his jaw to the left and his tongue to the right, they couldn't differentiate and wanted to move as a unit. As he kept exploring over several weeks, his mouth could open and close with a larger range, his chin could move without a quiver, and his tongue could move independently of his jaw. He also noticed a new dimension of spaciousness in the roof of his mouth and softness in his lips. And the movement of his breath seemed to fill his cranium as well as his chest. Was this what a relaxed jaw felt like? Although Tom's jaw was still one of his favorite places to store stress, he now knew how to let it go.

Relax Your Mind

After you've learned what relaxation looks and feels like in your body, you need to learn how to quiet your mind. Unless you're fatigued, injured, or medicated, the source for stress and tension is probably mental or emotional. When relaxation is your goal, your body is your ally and your wandering, busy, fretful mind is your challenge. This is compounded when you live in a complex world with a lot of distractions, uncertainties, and demands.

It's easy to understand how your head gets filled with rapid-fire images and nonstop chatter when it's constantly bombarded with stimuli and information. Like most people, your mind probably seems as if it has an agenda that resists relaxation. Even when you intend to de-stress using all of the strategies outlined earlier, your mind can undo everything in a millisecond. Even when you've finally relaxed your body at the end of the day, the demanding narrative in your mind can erupt with the details of your next vacation, your shopping list, or a troubling emotional/financial issue. As my client Joan observed, "It is like my head is a closet that's jammed full of stuff that keeps spilling out into my calm living room."

What is the state of your mind? Does it seem like it's filled with an endless stream of words, dialogues, images, memories, and imaginations? Does the loud, nonstop, nervous, insistent mental verbiage drown out your body awareness? Is there any room in there for peace and quiet? If your mind is in turmoil, your body can't be relaxed.

❀ Try This: Tense Thinking

Take a moment, close your eyes, and take a few breaths. Notice the space and shape of your body change with your inhale and exhale. What interior space is available for your breath? How deep and wide is your breath? How much of your body is filling and emptying? Now let your attention move from your body to a disturbing thought. For example:

- Your bank balance and/or projected earnings for this quarter

- A recent telephone call with a difficult customer, client, or family member

- The state of your health or the health of a loved one

- Tomorrow's complicated schedule or any unfinished business

- The political scene or turmoil of the world

When these thoughts entered the picture, did you feel your muscles contract? Did it seem harder to get a full breath? Remember, when your muscles tense up anywhere, they contract slightly everywhere. Your diminished breathing capacity is a reflection of the tension in your chest, ribs, and belly. This is the tension of a thought.

Years ago, scientists at UCLA used electromyography to measure the effects of stressful mental activity on the physical body. Their data showed how muscles throughout the body tighten slightly with any cognitive activity, stressful or not.[5]

....

5   Valerie V. Hunt, "Study of Structural Integration from Neuromuscular, Energy Field, and Emotional Approaches," Abstract 1977. www.anatomyfacts.com/Research/astudyof.pdf.

Recently, researchers found an interesting correlation: it's impossible to even entertain a negative or stressful thought if you're in a truly relaxed state.[6] Stress and relaxation just don't mix. Of course, the point here is not to stop thinking altogether but to be able to quiet your mind in order to de-stress and relax. Unfortunately, you may not have a clue how to do this. Unless you learn and practice a relaxation technique, you may be keyed up mentally and physically, waking or sleeping.

> *Margo.* *The only time Margo's mind seemed to quiet down was when she had a blazing headache. At her wits' end with the cycles of stress, medication, and debilitation, she feared there was no hope for someone so high-strung and hyper alert. Her body and her mind were at an impasse. When her naturopath suggested that she learn a relaxation technique, she eagerly pursued one technique after another to no avail— in fact they all seemed to only give her more to think about. Instead of approaching the process from the old perspective of cognition and performance, Margo's biggest challenge was to trust her body. When she came to me to learn my breath-centered meditation, we put her mind in the passenger's seat and her body in the driver's seat. After all, breathing is a bodily function. Changing the job descriptions helped her unravel the tangle of tension that'd held on for so long. Being "mindful" meant being "body-full" and "mind-empty." And, whenever stress threatened to accelerate into a headache, our girl knew how to pull into a rest stop and do some focused breathing.*

Four Relaxation Techniques

Like Margo discovered, the simplest way to quiet an overactive mind is to put your body in the driver's seat. There are some great body-centered ways to quiet your mind and relax your body. Add one to your self-care routine, give it some time, and see what happens. Developing relaxation skill gives *you* some control over the situation. Remember to be nonjudgmental and let the process be your teacher. Pretty soon you'll notice how your ability to relax changes the way you approach stress and the way stress affects you.

....

6   Charmaine Liebertz, "Want Clear Thinking? Relax," in *Scientific American Mind*, October 1, 2005, www.scientificamerican.com/article/want-clear-thinking-relax.

1. Body Breathing

From your body's perspective, it's clear that stress has a physical component. When stress becomes a lifestyle, amped-up physiology and muscle tension are a part of the package. Have you ever noticed how stress affects your breathing? One way to practice body-centered relaxation is to focus on the anatomical design of your breathing body. Not only will this help you relax, it will reset your baseline for stress. Follow these easy steps and your breathing body will help you relax:

1. Sit or lie down in a comfortable, quiet place.

2. Bring your full awareness to your breathing—exhale to inhale to exhale.

3. Let your ribs move freely. Soften any tension in your back, chest, and belly.

4. Don't overbreathe, just notice how it goes on its own.

5. Keep your focus on your body—bones and joints, organs, and soft tissues.

6. Whenever your attention wanders to word-thoughts, bring it back to your breathing body.

7. See how many full cycles you can string together.

As with any practice, you'll be a beginner before you feel any accomplishment. Be patient. Most people have a dominant holding pattern that restricts their breathing. As you reclaim the fullness of your breath, you may be releasing the stress of a lifetime. Don't project where you're going or get distracted by where you've been. Breathing is an anatomical function, and your body knows when it's right.

❀ Try This: Body Meditation

Here is a meditation I often use with my clients. Ask a friend to sit with you and read the following meditation out loud with a soft voice and measured cadence:

Close your eyes and tune in to your body breath. Place your hands lightly on your stomach and let your breath come here and soften the tension. Notice how this release frees up space so that your diaphragm and ribs can move a bit easier. Like the blinds on a window, feel your ribs pivot upward and downward with each inhale and exhale. Can you feel the gentle movement of your rib cage in your front and sides and back as well? Let the movement spill over to your shoulders and collarbone, tension does not hold back this easy flow. Keep your focus on your body and direct your moving body breath into your neck and head, pelvis and hips. This isn't a mental visualization—it is an actual physical feeling. Let your joints and tissues, your organs and sinews be gathered in to the gentle moving function of your breathing body. If any place feels stuck or stiff, let your breath get it moving. Let your breath be the medium that gathers all parts into the whole. Release worries, thoughts, and tension with each exhale. Open to peace and relaxation with each inhale. Linger here. This is you too.

At the beginning, a body meditation might only get as far as your belly and your attention might last two minutes. That's a good start. If you can stay focused for three to four breaths, you've accomplished something. Like any new learning, you'll be discovering a lot about your mind, emotions, habits, and assumptions as you go along. Each time you practice a body-centered relaxation technique, it'll teach you something and each time will be different. As your mind becomes more accustomed to the quiet, see if you can sit with your breathing body for fifteen to twenty minutes. Using the natural movement of breath to relax gives you a tool to decompress anytime you need it.

Tamara. Tamara seemed to get more agitated whenever she tried to quiet her mind. She not only felt anxious but judged herself for failing. The well-meaning encouragement from her friends felt like empty platitudes. I suggested that perhaps her first step would be a simple one: rather than take on a whole program and philosophy, why not start with what she knows best—her body? Her "practice" was to understand the anatomy of breathing (how the diaphragm, ribs, and lungs function) and check in with her breath periodically during the day to notice only what it was doing and not change anything. At first, she was startled to discover how often she actually held her breath. It seemed as if the flow of breath was sporadic and unpredictable no matter what she was doing, and she described it as "waking apnea." When Tamara fashioned her relaxation exercise as a study of breathing, it was easier for her mind to go along with the program. Setting time aside and following the protocol for body breathing, she finally discovered what relaxation felt like.

2. Focused Moving

You can practice a form of moving meditation anytime you do something and pay full attention to your body. No meandering thoughts or multitasking; no daydreaming or fantasizing. Let your mind step aside and be a curious observer as you focus squarely on the sensation and execution of any task. Centering your awareness in the action and sensation of your physical experience is a good way to quiet your mind and undermine the constant chatter of word-thoughts. However, it's likely that since your nonstop mind has run the show for so long, focused moving may be a skill you'll need to learn.

❀ Try This: Take Your Body for a Walk

Practice some focused moving the next time you go for a walk. As you go along, keep your full attention on feedback from your senses—*feel* your legs moving, your arms swinging; *smell* the scents in the air; *see* the play of light on the trees and buildings. Just notice it all and move on to noticing other physical things—the sound of children playing or the traffic nearby. Watch out for the temptation to go beyond simple, sensual observation. For instance, before you know it, the color of the sky sends your mind off thinking about a scarf you wanted to buy, or the smell of autumn leaves invites a plan for procuring firewood. Your mind is so accustomed to chatting and calculating that at first, it'll feel like trying to wrestle a greased pig (sorry, couldn't help myself). In addition to a pervasive habit, filling the airwaves with nonstop thinking is a way of avoiding physical discomfort and emotional feelings for some people. Don't be surprised if some personal growth opportunities accompany your moving meditation.

Did you notice how you were able to focus on your body for only a very short time before your mind intervened and demanded center stage? Just like breathing, it's impossible for your mind to attend to mind-talk and body-talk at the same time—it is one or the other. Once you get good at focused walking, try staying body-centered when you clean the house or walk the dog. Remember, the idea is not to evaluate, ruminate, or wax poetic about your perceptions. No matter what you're doing, you can relax a bit anytime you tune in to your moving body. This is a good way to keep centered and calm when going through stressful times.

> *Jonathan. Jonathan loved a challenge and strived to do his personal best. Several years after he got his MBA, he noticed that the demands of his job had become more stressful than exciting. Not only did the stress impede his fun, it also took the edge off his game. Even after a three-day weekend, he felt more anxious than relaxed. The spring in his step and a song in his heart had disappeared. Stress seemed to have filled the space where joy used to live. I suggested that he focus on his spacious body every morning on his walk to work. Doing his own version of a moving meditation, Jonathan used the natural flowing motion of his walking body to loosen the vise grip of discord in his hips and shoulders. Instead of looking at the ground, he looked to the horizon with his head up and shoulders back. Now with more space in his chest, his heart could open and he could breathe easier. Each easy swing of his arms and legs seemed to generate peace, confidence, and enthusiasm. When the day began with body-centered walking, a different Jonathan showed up for work. Learning to relax meant he had more clarity and more energy.*

3. Go Slow

Slowing down is a great strategy for managing stress. But it's also a great relaxation technique. Yet, like many people, the prospect of getting off the treadmill of go-go-go may seem like a radical, risky proposition. To really understand the effect of tempo on tension, you'll need to take the plunge and set up some "go slow sobriety." Understanding the way your body works is a good place to start. Did you know that your body is sourced in the natural world? Before machines and technology, the pace of living was aligned with the ebb and flow of the diurnal, seasonal, and physical world. Tasks took a certain amount of time and activities were seasonal. Today, you can do more at any time in less time, but just because you can doesn't mean you should. As every health professional (or auto mechanic, for that matter) can tell you, using a high gear nonstop will set you up for a breakdown.

One of the first things you may notice when you go slow is your addiction to the pace, adrenalin rush, and drama of going fast. Slowing down may seem flat and boring at first. It may bring up unpleasant feelings and memories, and consequently, you might not know what to do with yourself. If you encounter a *dependency issue*, tune in to your wise body to help you get off the *speed*. Let your curious mind follow the lead of your awake body. As you're eating breakfast, brushing hair or teeth, walking the dog, or wiping down the kitchen counter, let your body set the pace. Whenever you get physical, be physical. Match the muscle tension to the task. Match the pace to the activity. Moving too fast or too slow is a contraction. Moving in sync is relaxing. Studies have shown that slowing down reduces stress levels and increases efficiency and productivity.[7] Following are some occasions in your busy life to practice some *go slow* sobriety:

- Preparing/eating meals

- Attending to your hygiene

- Reading the paper/answering personal emails

- Walking anywhere

- Doing menial tasks, such as cleaning house or pumping gas

- Coming to a complete stop at a stop sign and taking one breath

Tune in to any in-between time and let your pace match the moment. Take time to taste the latte and smell the rose. Break the speeding habit and don't tailgate, eat on the run, or push the envelope. Remember, *adding speed to any task is adding another task*. Not only are you chopping vegetables, you're chopping vegetables and being fast. Not only are you packing a suitcase, you're packing a suitcase and doing it quickly. Not only are you shoveling snow, you're shoveling and rushing. You don't really get more done, you just add more tension/stress and perpetuate the speed habit.

---

7   Ray Williams, "Slowing Down Can Increase Productivity and Happiness," *Psychology Today*, June 17, 2014, www.psychologytoday.com/blog/wired-success/201406/slowing-down -can-increase-productivity-and-happiness-part-1.

❀ *Try This: Your Natural Pace*

Slowing it all down is not a new approach; it's a *natural* approach. Spend some time in nature and let it teach you about the fine art of going slow. Give yourself ten or fifteen minutes in a natural setting such as a beach, a park, or even your backyard. Simply sit quietly. Stop and listen and feel and get in sync with the tempo of the world around you. To do this, you'll need to transfer your attention from the rambling, rumbling of your mind to the sensual input of your body. Here's how:

- Relax your breath and let your senses open to the natural world

- Tune in to the pace and flow of the life around you

- Feel the gentle presence of air on your skin

- Hear the sound between sounds

- Observe the flight of a butterfly or the ripples of wind on water

- Let your body be an integral part of the surroundings

- Invite your mind to be sensual

When you hear the chorus of birdsong serenading from the canopy overhead or feel the freshness of the air after a storm or smell the sweet perfume of springtime, you're in the poetry of the moment. Aligning your body with the cadence of the natural world creates a baseline for relaxation. It's the speed your body knows in its primitive core. The intensity of your schedule and obligations mean nothing here. Let yourself linger, in sync with nature, for one more birdsong, one more breath. Anytime you need a re-minder, there's always a little bit of nature close at hand.

When you learn how to decelerate your pace to match each activity, you're able to be in the moment. To go slow doesn't mean going *too* slow. It's about paying attention and getting in sync. Walking with a toddler, washing your body, putting the groceries away, running along the beach, weeding the garden, and avoiding an accident have their own perfect pace. If you go too slowly, you miss the mark. If you try to speed up, you'll just increase tension and decrease attention/accuracy/efficiency. Can you feel it? Like most people, speeding things up is habitual and unconscious, not to mention it is also cultural. Why do you think they call it a rat race? If you slow it down, you can step off the wheel and get wherever you're going with more awareness and ease and a lot less stress. Take another minute to sit at lunch, linger in bed, or pause before work. When you slow down to your natural pace, you can live in each micromoment; you have more time rather than less and a whole lot more enjoyment.

4. Lighten Up

You have a choice between seeing your day in colorful tones or in blacks and grays. Sure, stuff goes on in your life and the world around you that can feel immediate, profound, and sometimes tragic. But piling a message of fear, despair, and unhappiness on your body is way too cumbersome and is also unproductive, stressful, and unhealthy. As you'll learn in chapter 6, feelings move through like the weather. A storm gathers and then passes through. When an emotional expression gets stuck in your body, you lose the option of moving on. If you plant fear in your stomach, it's hard to take a fresh breath. If you wear sorrow on your shoulders, it's hard for them to shake freely with laughter. One way to loosen up and lighten up is to practice being consciously happy. Curiously, you don't actually have to *feel* happy in order for it to work.

Research has shown that performative merriment alters moods.[8] For years, actors have known that getting into character really meant that character was getting into them. In real life, they became grouchy when they were playing a grump; disrespectful when they were playing a misogynist; goofy when they were playing a joker. Their experience has now been explained in the laboratory. Biochemists have validated that acting in a comedy enhances immune function/lowers stress hormone levels and acting in a tragedy depresses immune function/increases stress hormones.[9] In addition, lightening up a bit is a good way to generate positive feelings, change your thoughts, and de-stress your body.

....

8   Erin Brodwin, Jessica Orwig, and Dina Spector, "How to Feel Happier, According to Neuroscientists and Psychologists," in *Business Insider,* July 11, 2017. uk.businessinsider.com/how-feel-happy-happier-better-2017-7.html.

9   Judith Ohikuare, "How Actors Create Emotions: A Problematic Psychology," in *The Atlantic,* March 10, 2014. www.theatlantic.com/health/archinve/2014/03/how-actors-create-emotions-a-problematic-psychology/284291/.html.

❀ Try This: How Does Happy-Sad-Mad Feel?

Test out the research in your own body. In the privacy of your bedroom or bathroom, imagine you're an actor playing the role of an angry person. How would this look, sound, and feel? As you contract your muscles into the shape and expression of anger, do *you* feel slightly angry as well? As you contract your throat to say a few words in an angry tone, does your chest tighten? Is it harder to breathe and see the bright side of things? Now imagine you are an actor playing the role of a person in love walking on the sunny side of the street. How does this affect your body and mood? Where did the anger go? What about fear, frustration, sorrow? Can you feel how these acting roles can get into your body?

There's actually a laughing therapy based on studies that show you get the very same psychological and physiological benefits whether it's authentic or not.[10] You can feel it happen. No matter how ridiculous or contrived it may seem, take a few minutes to be happy any time and notice how the tenor of the day changes. As you sit at your desk, shift a scowl to a smile and see if it elevates your mood. Try skipping a bit the next time you're out for a walk. Sing out loud with the radio while driving in the car. The power of the positive—thought, expression, word, and gesture—not only affects your own physiology but seems to influence the people around you as well. You've probably experienced the uplifting effect of a cheery sales clerk or caring friend.

Maurice. When Maurice first tried the "be happy" approach, he had to push through some serious tension in his cheeks to achieve a full-on smile. It'd been a long time since he felt any overt reason for happiness, and it was alarming to feel how the stress and tension had set up like concrete in his face. No wonder he felt tired and hopeless all the time. In order to change the way he "faced" the future, Maurice needed to work on the present moment. Strange as it may seem, he needed to learn how to smile again. Each morning, Maurice stood in front of the mirror and took a few minutes to pull his cheeks into a big smile. Even though he was just acting, it was hard not to chuckle a bit when he saw that goofy grin. In a very short time, the concrete started to break up and the smile began to feel familiar. Lightening up his demeanor, Maurice felt less burdened and more lighthearted and relaxed.

....

10   Ryan Howes, "Laughter in Therapy," in *Psychology Today*, Dec. 31, 2013. www.psychologytoday .com/blog/in-therapy/201312/laughter-in-therapy.

✿ *Try This: How Do You Face the World?*

If you spend time in serious pursuits in a pretty serious world, chances are being lighthearted and relaxed aren't your default mode. If your muscles gravitate to frowning, wincing, or scowling, your very expression can stress you out. Just let your face tell you about it. As you stand in front of a mirror, close your eyes and bring your expression to what feels normal. Then open your eyes and really see how you're facing the world. Does your reflection look peaceful, delighted, loving, or hopeful? Or, do you see puzzlement, concern, grief, anger, disgust, or struggle? Like Maurice, are the lines and wrinkles shaped by the stresses of yesterday and worries for tomorrow? Close your eyes again and let your expression soften. Think of something delightful or endearing and open your eyes to take a look. Do you look less stressed, more attractive? Do you look younger? Do you feel younger, happier, more relaxed? You may be surprised to learn that it takes more muscle effort to frown than it does to smile.

Body breathing, focused moving, slowing down, and lightening up are four ways to let go of stress and relax. All of them will quiet your mind chatter and change your outlook. All of them will activate your happy physiology and help you be more relaxed no matter what you're doing. If stress is cumulative, relaxation is as well. Once you figure this out, it's your choice. Your body knows the difference and it can help you make the difference. Like anything new, getting good at relaxation is a learning process. Once you find the techniques that work, your practice will be the teacher. This is not just a glib statement. Stay with it and you'll know what it means. It takes time to master the art of relaxation.

✿ *Explore: Letting Go and Holding On*

Once you decide to do something about stress and learn how to relax, the process has begun. In your Body Wisdom journal, describe what you've discovered about yourself and your body from the stress strategies and relaxation exercises in this chapter. List the ways your body carries stress and why you need to learn to relax. Describe the personalized, body-centered relaxation technique that works best for you, and make a commitment to practice over the next five days … or weeks, months, or even years. Describe your day-to-day experience in your journal as you go along. Simply observe and record. The experience of being and staying quiet is novel and challenging in our culture. Just taking off the straightjacket of tension and clearing your mind of word-thoughts clutter can reveal some provocative insights. Some things you might notice:

- Resistance, avoidance, procrastination, and distraction patterns
- Disquieting discomforts of the flesh
- Persistent interference of the monkey mind
- Tension comes into the body when the mind takes over
- When your mind takes over, your body disappears
- Keeping your focus on your body quiets your mind
- Emotional expression (sigh, moan, sob, shiver) helps muscles relax
- Clarity, energy, and inspiration that follows your practice

Observe what comes up and ask yourself why. Then, write down your insights. Taking the time to feel and release muscle tension can tell you a lot about your relationship with your body. Don't be surprised if relaxation techniques are easier in theory than practice. Taking time to relax can feel like swimming against prevailing currents. At first it might feel daunting to set aside even five minutes to clear your mind of stimulating and re-stimulating images, feelings, and thoughts. Don't be discouraged; be persistent. Over time, your relaxation practice will link you up with the sensible undercurrent of the natural world—the rhythms of the day, the song of the birds, the flow of the seasons, and the comfort of your measured breathing. It will change the way you live in the world.

Check out other strategies to help you let go and relax. Classes in yoga, tai chi, and meditation are designed to help you slow down and de-stress. A massage, facial, manicure, pedicure, or simply a soak in a warm bath will help you feel good and relax. Listening to soft music or a guided meditation CD, eating dinner with friends, knitting a sweater, stroking your pet, or taking a vacation are great ways to counter stress and relax. That said, it may seem at times that no matter how many things you try or techniques you practice, it is impossible to crack the hold of tension on your body-mind. If your efforts only seem to create frustration and the tension-pain-tension goes around and around, you may be up against a wall of entrenched stress that needs professional care. Dietary changes, acupuncture, and herbal remedies in addition to physician-prescribed anti-anxiety and/or anti-depression medications can break negative cycles, give you relief, and support your body's ability to let go of tension.

Your growing awareness of your body will help you and your health practitioner construct an effective therapeutic team. Talk therapy, dance therapy, psychodrama, and hands-on body therapies are highly effective for interrupting anxiety, hypertension, and other stress related conditions. My particular bias is that if something's in the body, it needs to be addressed in the body. If you and your therapist listen, the body will reveal what is ready to be seen as well as the necessary progression for healing.

Make no mistake, taking care of stress and learning how to relax is a worthy endeavor. Everything you put into it will pay off in dividends every day for the rest of your life. Stress strategies and relaxation practices are never more important than when you face an intense event like divorce, loss, any big change, birth, death, illness, or a catastrophic event. Any personal crisis related to health, finances, relationships, creativity, or emotions can set your body on high alert. Yet as you know, unless you're *actually* fleeing the tiger, the physiology of fight-or-flight is bad for your health and only gets in the way. Just think of a time when you spent a restless night going over and over an issue or event. Wouldn't it have been helpful to know some of these stress strategies and relaxation techniques to help you out at 4:00 am? Wouldn't it be an asset to know how to calm down and center before the next big presentation, final exam, or family meeting? Wouldn't it be prudent to have some of these essentials in place before a health crisis or unexpected emergency?

Pascal. Pascal was in the throes of a tricky real estate transaction. Not only were her future plans at stake, but so was a lot of money. Her mind was in high gear and she couldn't relax enough to get to sleep. In desperation, she remembered her relaxation practice. Instead of letting her mind spin out thinking about "what if" and "if only," she focused on her breath and her body. Instead of going outside herself, she went inside and followed the breath moving her belly and ribs. Going around her mind and through her body was soothing and reassuring. Rather than all the drama and details, her body affirmed: "all is in right order, everything comes in its own time and, no matter what, life goes on." At that very moment, her head and neck succumbed to the gentle rocking of her breath. Pascal fell into a deep, restful sleep. The next morning, she had the fresh perspective and mental acuity to make decisions that were in her best interest.

Stress, hypertension, and lifelong holding patterns can act as roadblocks to knowing and living in your body. In order to find and use your body wisdom, these obstacles need to be removed. This chapter has helped you identify and change your template of tension. Take the techniques, strategies, and practices you've learned and put them in your personal toolbox. Chances are there'll be an opportunity to use one or two every day to dismantle some lifelong habits of overreacting and overmuscling. Like Pascal discovered, the tools you acquire today can get you out of a jam in stressful times. And, over the long run, they may even save your life.

Now that you have the body basics covered and know how to relax, you're ready to explore the exciting topics of body-oriented healing, emotional intelligence, intimacy, intuition, and spiritual meaning.

Five
Healing

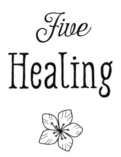

As a good steward of your body, health is your ultimate goal. Usually, awareness and basic self-care are all you need to stay healthy and whole. It's pretty simple to understand that poor eating, sleeping, and exercising habits along with less-than-optimal stress and time management set the scene for poor health. Yet even with the best practices in place, illness and injury can just happen. Now, instead of options and optimism, you encounter limitation and discomfort. The return to full function and comfort is a specific puzzle that needs to be solved. In order to get the guidance you need and to do the job of healing, you need to reorder your priorities and put your body front and center.

Even if you feel confident of your body's innate wisdom, it can be challenging to trust it when you feel weak, brittle, cranky, and uncomfortable. When you're not feeling well, the simplest things can seem daunting or overwhelming physically *and* emotionally. Let's face it: a minor cold can put you off your stride; a seasonal flu can stop you in your tracks; and something life-threatening can throw you over the edge. Whenever health and mobility are diminished, it's natural to feel a degree of uncertainty and fear. Don't be surprised if your positive outlook disappears and some old habits of denial and distortion resurface. For instance, when you're faced with a health issue, is your first impulse to doubt your body? Do you want to flee to a specialist or fight your symptoms?

Do you freeze up and hope it all goes away? Observing and addressing these baseline impulses is part of the healing process.

The Span of Wellness

Your body's health status is never static. Depending on variables of stress and circumstance, your physical function, vitality, and strength are constantly balancing and rebalancing. This constantly changing process is ongoing, subtle, and taken for granted. Every once in a while, for one reason or another, the balance tilts too much or you encounter a roadblock where getting back on track requires something more—more time, more input, and more commitment. By now you've probably experienced this fluctuating health dynamic more than once.

Have you ever been sailing along, on top of your game, when something shifts and you find yourself in stormy seas? To get back on an even keel, your first question might be, "How did this happen?" Maybe your self-care routines were sidelined by laziness or distraction; maybe stress or worry undermined your good intentions; maybe it was an accident or a virus or something in the gene pool; maybe it was in the stars; maybe it was just part of the up-and-down cycle. Whatever the cause, when your body needs healing, it's asking you to pay attention and recommit yourself to wellness. Whether you're dealing with a head cold, sprained ankle, or a serious illness, it's all part of living in a physical world. Anytime you need to heal, your curious mind will discover new things about your smart body.

Most of this book is dedicated to the practices and perspectives of how to be healthy and stay healthy. So far, you've learned to trust your body as a reliable partner when it comes to paying attention, showing up, learning new things, and designing a self-care program that works. Now it's time to trust your body and let it be an active participant in your own healing. This chapter focuses on what to do when your body needs help and *you* need to be the adult in charge.

Changing Your Mind about Your Body

When you're not strong and healthy, it's easy to think your body has let you down. Even a brief cold can precipitate thoughts of weakness and vulnerability. When healing lasts longer than a day or two and follows a complicated course, you may think that your body is not your ally. It is not uncommon for people dealing with chronic conditions, long-term illness and trauma to distance themselves from their body altogether. After all, it's easy to think that the body is the problem … and even the enemy. Here, the philosophical argument that *you are not your body* comes in handy. Consider that if you're not occupying the premises, you're not showing up for the healing journey.

In order to access all of your resources, you may need to change your mind about your body. If your body is listening in, what is it hearing? Consider the message you'd like to convey and make sure your thoughts and words communicate steadfast trust, gratitude, hope, and love.

What's Your Assignment?

You can probably identify the difference between the symptoms of a cold, allergy, or sugar overload. You know how to get your body back in balance. If you fall down and cut your leg, you have a pretty good idea whether simple bandaging or stitches are necessary. With input from various health professionals, the popular press, wellness websites, and your grandmother, you're pretty well versed in basic care and repair. Yet, even a simple healing assignment can teach you something new if you use your body wisdom.

The healing assignment gets a bit more complicated when it involves a sprained ankle, gallbladder surgery, or recovery from a fender bender. This is not an everyday balance/rebalance situation. It'll take a little more time, attention, and trust. You'll need help from professionals, family, and friends. You've left the "same ol', same ol'" and entered into new territory where the route to healing includes patience, humility, and rehabilitation. Getting onboard and doing your part will help you feel empowered and speed your recovery. Perhaps, along the way, you'll meet your inner healer.

When your assignment involves something major such as a genetic complication, autoimmune disease, cancer, major accident, or recovery from addiction, you'll be on a healing journey that can last a long time and change the way you live in the world. Now is the time to dig deep, be diligent, and assemble a good team. Keep in mind that no matter how debilitated and dependent you might feel, your role is far from passive. *You are the key player on the team.* You'll need to show up, ask for help, and receive it graciously. You'll need to learn about your condition, participate in the protocols, and get comfortable living on the edge. Now more than ever, you'll need to trust your body wisdom and let it be your guide. As the journey unfolds, your healing will touch every part of who you are.

When you have any healing assignment, large or small, your smart body is a primary resource, an indispensable partner. This chapter will show you how to tune in to your body and listen to its wisdom. Now's the time to put everything you've learned to the test: What's going on? Is there a deeper agenda? Where do you need help? What help is working? Talk to your body and listen to your body-talk. Remember that healing happens from the inside out. Let your body be the focal point and use this valuable asset for healing.

Three Steps to Healing

The first four chapters helped you find your smart body, get inside, and take care of the basics. You've had some experience with the symbolic language of body-talk. Listening to your sentient, intelligent body has helped you set up effective self-care routines and changed your stress profile. You've enhanced your understanding and changed the way you think about yourself. This new body-centered awareness will help you be an empowered, conscious participant in your own healing. Here are eight body-wise ways to help you participate in the healing process.

Get a Grip!

Regardless of the particulars, anytime your health is compromised, your body's telling you to *do* something. Don't delay, deny, or panic, but do *get a grip*. This is the time to return to the source and listen to your feelings, mind, and body to set the course for healing.

Listening to your feelings means getting perspective and taking a moment to assess the situation. Many health practitioners believe that the body is more vulnerable to illness and injury when the emotions are triggered or the mind is preoccupied. Could there be a relationship between your behavior or mindset and your current health issue? Could there be a connection between feeling overstressed, overworked, out of ease, and disease? Could there be a connection between injury and a feeling of distraction or a lack of focus? Even if you think it dropped out of the blue, looking at your health issue through a wide-angle lens will give you the full picture. This doesn't mean getting stuck in the "woulda/shoulda/coulda" blame game. It means acknowledging the whole as-signment and getting on with it.

Certainly when you get sick or injured, it's easy to feel resistance, denial, fear, re-sentment, and vulnerability. When you feel weaker, shakier, and less capable of tackling even mundane chores, you need to change your plans and ask for help. And even asking can bring up feelings of uncertainty and anxiety. Living with fewer options and more in-convenience can bring up feelings of anger and resentment. Listen to and process these feelings. They're not a distraction—they're a part of your healing. *Getting a grip* means embracing the whole picture and staying on track. Doing this at the front end will save a lot of energy and give you the confidence to proceed and succeed.

> *Khalila. Khalila fell off her horse and injured her hip. Before it was completely healed, she reinjured it doing yoga. Even with the best professional help, her healing had taken longer than she expected and an old feeling of impatience was making her doubt her body. Her deepest fear was that she'd never ride again. To get a grip and break the stranglehold of negative feelings, she began to listen, express, and honor her feelings. Stopping in at this place of fear and sorrow for a moment was a part of the healing journey. Instead of perpetuating her doubt, this emboldened her confidence. Even though her movement and comfort were still restricted, she trusted her strong body to find its way to full recovery.*

You can't get on with your healing assignment when you're indulging old routines of self-doubt and self-judgment. Much of this chapter is about how *you* factor into the picture. Healing isn't just about the injury or illness—it's about you. If you hear even the faintest whisper of "I brought this on myself," "I must have needed this," or "I'm never going to get well," it's imperative to dig deeper and heal the underlying blame, shame, anger, resentment, sorrow, and fear. (To find out more about this, see the next chapter, on emotional embodiment.) This is your opportunity to change the old messaging of despair, fear, and self-deprecation. Exploring the emotional precursors to illness and injury means letting the world of symbol, self-talk, and metaphor enhance your heal-ing, not fuel your blame. Remember, if you want your uber-smart body to help you heal, you need to sign the "hold harmless" agreement.

As you step back to observe the symptoms and effect of what's happening, you may be uncovering an important piece of your healing puzzle. Your health team needs to have this information in order to come up with an accurate diagnosis and an effective course for recovery. How do *you* fit in to the picture? This personal information will help them help you. Did the stress or circumstance of the past few weeks (or months or year) set you up for distraction or dis-ease? Addressing the whole person can be just as important as stitching up the wounded part.

❋ Explore: Emotional Intake Interview

Your emotional physiology is not only a precursor to illness but also to injury. Perhaps what you're feeling is directly linked to how you feel. As you discovered in previous chapters, emotions have an effect on your biochemistry, attitude, and performance. When you feel sad, frustrated, worried, or fatigued, it influences your focus, balance, and coordination. An Emotional Intake interview highlights where you've been, how you got here, and what needs to change. It'll help you *get a grip*, show up, and be ready to do your part. Here are some pointed questions to ask:

- What was going on with my body/mind before I got sick/hurt?

- What was going on in my personal/professional life?

- What was happening in the news?

- What was I feeling and why?

Write out the timeline, your feelings, insights, and discoveries in your Body Wisdom journal. Flesh out the story. Ask the part of your body that's sick or injured to weigh in. How does it relate to or embody your personal and external circumstances? How might the injury or illness reflect the course of events? Keep your attention in your body and pause long enough to hear the answer—*from your body.* Set aside some space in your journal to add more insights as time goes on.

Charles. *Charles's fingers had been going numb for some time. Once he had a full medical workup, it was ascertained that his slumping posture was adversely affecting the nerves running down his arms. It would take some effort on his part, but his doctor was confident that with time and good physical therapy, Charles could avoid surgery. Rather than see this news as a positive prognosis, Charles felt depressed. Taking the time to do an Emotional Intake interview made it clear that losing the feeling in his fingers was one more loss in a string of losses. Just over the past year he had retired, his mother had died, and he had lost his sense of purpose. Looking at the mind-body connection, Charles got a laugh when he realized that his numb fingers matched the way he'd been "handling" his losses. Perhaps, before the hangdog could become a happy dog, he needed to let go of his grief and anger. Seeing the big picture helped Charles get a grip on his healing assignment.*

Filling out the Emotional Intake interview doesn't mean your situation is psychosomatic or you intended to get sick/injured. "Stuff" happens. Khalila did injure her hip; Charles did have bad posture. However, both needed to *get a grip* and come to terms with the psychological context and their feelings about their physical circumstances. Does your current health issue churn up some old judgments and assumptions about not being well and needing help? Do you feel regret, frustration, doubt, sorrow, anger, or fear? Do you feel vulnerable, uncertain, out of control, awkward, needy, impatient, resentful, anxious, apologetic, isolated, or abandoned? Listen to your feelings, give them expression, and take your first step on the healing journey.

Listening to your mind often means changing your mind. Changing your mind means paying attention when you get sick or injured and all the old tapes and attitudes resurface. Even when you're just slightly off your game, listen in on the internal dialogue and you might be surprised by what you hear. Toxic beliefs and obstructive attitudes often get triggered when you feel crummy. Your mind can concoct all kinds of unsavory scenarios when your body feels immobilized, hurt, tired, scared, anxious, or sad. You could be holding on to some beliefs or judgments about your body that are counterproductive to healing. For instance, some people believe that paying attention to distress, unease, or uncertainty will only make things worse. Others believe that letting the body be comforted and soothed is akin to coddling a spoiled child. And still others believe that they're not really their body anyway so it doesn't make a difference. Listen to the chatter and clean up the subtext so your mind can be onboard for healing.

✿ *Explore: Clean Up the Chatter*

When your body's sick or injured, its pleas for help might be drowned out by negative self-talk. In order to *get a grip* and get on with healing, you'll need to listen to your mind and clean up the chatter. This isn't a diversion; it's part of the healing. Get out your Body Wisdom journal and continue your Emotional Intake interview. Write down all the ideas and feelings that being sick/injured has brought up.

- What do you really think about your current situation?

- Is it your fault?

- Does it reflect on your character or worth?

- What are some family attitudes/beliefs that add to the context?

It's important to *see* the mess before you clean it up. Root out anything that feels or sounds negative, distracting, and judgmental. Write a positive script to help rather than hinder your healing intentions. Instead of a sign of weakness, maybe your injury is a sign of a strong body that knows when it needs time out to recuperate and repair. Instead of a pointless detour, your injury may be taking you exactly where you need to go on the path of life. Your goal in this exploration is to align the dominant message in your mind with the power and potential of your body. Your body is listening to your thoughts and words, so make sure they're on track for healing.

Listening to your mind when your body is hurting is an opportunity to change the way you relate to your body, yourself, and the world. It helps you be mindful throughout your healing journey. Even this season's flu can give you just enough pause to confirm your regard, love, and trust for your body. If your healing takes longer, the opportunity to change your mindset about your body can be so deep and profound that it's truly transformative.

Sally. When Sally's doctor told her that her abdominal pain was Crohn's disease, she needed to reset her thinking in order to accept the diagnosis and move forward. Although Sally knew how to give to others, she didn't know how to give to herself. Listening to her mind was like listening to a constant broadcast of judgment and criticism. She blamed her body for being flawed and felt worthless and hopeless. In order to get a grip, Sally needed to rewrite her own "bill of rights" and receive the help she'd so generously given to others. Once she let her body be entitled to time for healing and rebalance, her attitude changed. The old adage "for everything there is a season" gave her a positive reframe to apply her considerable capabilities and compassion on the homefront. Now was the time to dedicate herself to a very worthy cause—learning how to receive.

Jake. On weekends, Jake loved to take to the trails on his mountain bike. Several months ago, he hit a rock and catapulted over his handlebars, seriously injuring his shoulder. Once the surgical repairs were done, he found himself facing months of rehab and the boredom of physical therapy. While his body was trying to heal, his mind was replaying the movie over and over again looking for fault and blame. For Jake, accidents didn't just happen. In order to free up his energy and change his mindset, Jake needed to dislodge his "if only" theme and lose the judgment. He needed to change his perspective. "Why didn't I see the obstacle?" and "I shouldn't have been daydreaming" were about looking backward. In order to rebuild and trust the process, Jake used his mind power to deliver the message, "You need to climb the mountain and face the obstacles in order to ride down again." From this point of view, his rehab program looked like a good way to get even better at his sport.

Both Sally and Jake used their physical situation to *get a grip* and change their mindset. After the diagnosis and setting of the bones, the real work of healing begins. This is an opportunity to enlist the positives and reframe the negatives. In order to get your body back on track, you'll need all your energy zeroed in on physical healing. Listen to your mind and make sure it's aligned with the task at hand.

Listening in gives you a powerful way to elicit your deepest healing potential. Your overt symptoms tell you more than where your body needs to rebalance. Symptoms can also tell you where your body-mind-spirit needs realignment. Listen to your body and hear the subtext. For instance, your inflamed sore throat may have a strep infection *and* it may be holding onto some angry words. Your sore ankle may be sprained *and* it may represent the painful steps you're taking. As corny as it seems, in the world of your body, symptoms are often quite literal. In this manner, the front side represents what is in front of you. Your heart is your heart. Your feet are your support and understanding. If you invite your body to weigh in on its own terms, it can help you get a grip and answer the questions "What's going on?" "What do you need?" and "What do you want to tell me?"

🌸 *Try This: Is Your Body Telling You Something?*

Listening to your body might reveal a subtext in your health situation. In order to heal from the inside out, it's imperative to address imbalance, dis-ease, and distortion on all levels. As an orthopedic surgeon casually remarked, "I never knew a person with a broken bone who didn't need a 'break'!" Think of all the body related phrases you use such as *pain in the neck, shoulder the burden, a leg up, brought to your knees, hold your tongue,* and so on. Could one of these be a precursor of your current health situation? Think of your problem and use your imagination. Following are some intriguing examples:

- If your stomach is upset, it may be saying, "I don't have the stomach for this conversation (or relationship, career, confrontation) right now."

- If your neck seizes up, it may be communicating "something/someone is a pain in the neck" or "I'm sticking my neck too far out."

- If your back aches, it might mean "something is holding me back," "I have no backup," or "I'm backed up against a wall."

- If your shoulder hurts, perhaps the message is "I'm shouldering too much," or "I've had to shoulder through a difficult time."

Listen to your body—it knows what it's talking about! The very symptoms of your health situation can reveal a powerful asset for healing—the mind-body connection. Did you know that all languages the world over have vernacular phrases linking physical and situational discomfort? It's a universal understanding that an unresolved problem is a *pain in the neck* or an unsettling situation has the *stomach in knots.* Check out how body-talk helped Pam and Leonard get a grip on the whole picture and heal their attitude as well as their bodies.

Pam. Every time Pam reinjured her right foot, she powered through it. Her will was driving the program and all she cared about was job performance and getting through the door of success. When she listened to her body, she realized that instead of walking through the door, she'd been trying to kick it open! Now, not a single step could be taken (quite literally) toward her goals or her healing until she re-evaluated her approach. Her body was demonstrating the old adage "the more you push, the greater the resistance." In order to heal her body, Pam needed to move toward success with body-mind-spirit, not just ambition. Learning about gait and timing and cooperative interaction were helpful for her career as well as her body. When she walked back into the workplace with a new understanding, her sure-footedness carried a message of strength, resiliency, and confidence. Her body-mind-spirit were in sync with her goals and her injury had delivered the perfect win-win scenario.

Leonard. Leonard's chest hurt when he breathed. His cardiologist determined that the problem was musculoskeletal rather than organic. Through yoga, meditation, and massage, he was able to relax and relieve his discomfort. In addition, these practices gave him the space to quiet down and listen to his body. When he asked, "What's going on? What do you need? What do you want to tell me?" his body had a clear answer. His heart wasn't in his work anymore; he needed to reassign much of his workload and use his considerable talents promoting projects that reflected his core values. Instead of spending days doing heartless tasks, he now had time to pursue matters of the heart. Could this issue of the heart have been the true essence of Leonard's health problem?

❀ *Try This: Find the Gift*

Listening to your symbolic body is empowering, as well as illuminating. It'll help you identify the subtext of your situation and it will also help you look for and *find the gift*. Take a moment right now and get high above the earthly details of flesh and bone to see the whole trajectory of your journey. Embrace all of the aspects (your situation, feelings, mind chatter, learning curve) and see where you've been and what you've learned. Even the shortest healing journey has a gift for you. Look for it and find it. Use the rich language and images of metaphor and fairy tale to let the victim become the warrior and wake up the sleeping princess. Remember, symbol and story are a doorway to your nonverbal body. When you find the gift, acknowledge it. Say to yourself, "Without taking this journey, I would never have _____," or "This journey has taught me about _____." Perhaps your healing assignment has made you aware of the importance of how you think about your body. Perhaps it has been the vehicle to experience the presence of spirit in the flesh. Perhaps it has taught you about the interconnectedness of all life. The gift becomes more substantial when you put it in words. Anytime you can see a greater good, you give your healing body a boost of hope; any time you can find deeper meaning, you give your mind a boost of confidence. So often at the end of a healing journey, clients have confided, "the gifts I've received make the arduousness/ pain/turmoil/effort of the journey worth it."

Cleaning up and clearing out the disruptive and distracting feelings, thoughts, and attitudes will help you get a grip and get onboard. Changing your mindset, shifting your perspective, and finding the gift have put your feet squarely on the path to healing. Now, your "inner healer" is ready to get proactive.

Get Proactive!

Once you have an idea of what's going on, it's time for the second step in your healing program: getting proactive and assembling your team. For your healing situation, you may have a variety of treatment possibilities from allopathic to acupuncture to naturopathy to energy healing. If you break a bone, you'll want to see an orthopedic doctor with follow-up physical therapy. For a digestive ailment, you might see an internist or a naturopath to check for imbalances or infections in your gut. If you've suffered a trauma, in addition to the physical repair, you might want a somatic (body-oriented) therapist on the team to address your psychology. It's not in the purview of this book to suggest which course or combination of health modalities is appropriate for you or your situation. Being proactive means showing up with all you've got and doing your part.

When your body needs healing and you need help, it's tempting to give away your authority and assign the responsibility to caregivers and professionals. But, being *proactive* doesn't mean sitting back and turning your health over to professionals, protocols, and pharmaceuticals. Being a part of the team and doing your part has a measurable effect on the course and scope of your healing. Just being proactive can be a reassuring antidote to confusion, doubt, fear, and worry.

If you show up with all you've got and address the healing at hand, you just might heal much more than your body. Following are some good ways to get proactive by making it personal, walking your talk, being honest, and changing the story.

Make it personal. When the job is yours and your assignment is to get well, healing gets personalized. Sometimes this entails researching on your own and tracking down everything you can find about your condition; sometimes it means following a regimen that's difficult and unpleasant; and sometimes it means delving into your history, personality, and feelings. One thing is for sure—when you choose to show up wholeheartedly and make it personal, you'll learn a lot about yourself in the process. Life as usual changes, if only for twenty-four hours. Whether short- or long-term, healing is an intimate experience. If you encounter resistance, it's your resistance. If emotion comes up, it's your emotion. If you feel pain, it's your pain. And when you have a breakthrough and resolve an issue, it's your success. Whenever you learn something new, find your power, and recover your health, it's a personal triumph. Whenever you veer away from radiant well-being and find yourself on a healing journey, your priorities need to become very personal.

Walk your talk. Remember how your personal sound bites and outdated beliefs got in the way when you needed to get a grip? Your words can undermine your intentions at any stage on your healing journey. Negative self-talk is always counterproductive. Listen to the words you use as well as what you say to and about yourself. Are these words about strength, support, and hope? In order to truly walk your talk for healing, you may need to change the message.

On a healing journey, language is important. Your words and thoughts represent your beliefs. Pay attention—if a particular belief phrase pops up, be curious and check it out. Where did this phrase come from? Was it family members, educators, media marketing, religious teachings, or the culture at large? What do the words exactly mean? Do they match your intentions to heal and be healthy? Perhaps you have a choice phrase or two to add to the following list:

- Sickness implies weakness.

- No pain, no gain.

- I did something to deserve this and God (or the universe) is punishing me.

- I always get the short end of the stick.

- One step forward, two steps back.

If your body is listening (and it is), what messages do these convey? In order to make sure the language you use is supporting the goal of healing, replace every negative with an empowering statement, such as: "Every breakdown is a breakthrough," or "my body is designed to heal." Don't be surprised by the sudden appearance of self-deprecating or self-doubting self-talk when your body gets weak, injured, or sick. Just do something about it! Being proactive means getting your internal dialogue on your side for healing.

❀ Try This: Brushing Off Negatives

Take a proactive approach—brush the unproductive messages off your body as if they were dust. This gesture interrupts the negative and creates an opening for a positive that truly supports your healing intentions. Take three breaths to set the new positive message in place. No matter how corny or contrived this may seem, brushing off the old and breathing in the new is an effective self-hypnosis technique. Below are some ways clients have reframed their messages:

- "I am such a klutz" (brush) to "My body knows what to do" (breathe).

- "I have weak genes" (brush) to "I have a long lineage to back me up" (breathe).

- "Why me?" (brush) to "I have something to learn" (breathe).

Listen to what you're saying. Do you hear fear and negativity underscore a casual comment or harmless, homey saying? Ferret out the negative (brush) and replace them with the positive (breathe). Don't underestimate the importance of walking your talk. A variant of the principle of magnetic attraction is at play here. What you think, say, or believe will determine what you'll energize and attract, and this is true for negative as well as positive self-talk. Check out how different they feel in your body! Quantum healing theory suggests that giving your voice to a statement and your thought to an image is a powerful resource for healing.[11]

Get real. Addressing the emotional overlay of your health breakdown is as important as rest, recuperation, and rehab. Simply being waylaid or inconvenienced by a health issue is enough to make you mad, sad, or scared. To further complicate things, a healing journey has the potential to unearth some old, unresolved issues of vulnerability and self-worth. Not only do emotions get triggered, they might also have been a factor before your health breakdown. Look at your Emotional Intake interview. Before your illness or injury, were you under extra stress? Were you unhappy or disturbed? As you discovered in the chapter on stress and relaxation, your body is the place where you feel, hold, and express your emotions. If you are stuck or repressed, your emotions can turn toxic and actually make you sick.

The physiological connection between your emotional state and physical stress has a direct impact on your ability to focus and function. Here's a layman's picture of how this works: When feelings get bottled up, they create a sort of emotional logjam. With no release, pressure builds up over time. Your management strategies (denial, diversion, distraction) can't hold your emotions off forever and the resulting flood escapes through an emotional or a physical breakdown. The blocked energy simply must be channeled somewhere. What if getting hurt or sick was your body's way to release a back load of emotional residue? Even if it wasn't the cause, it makes sense to *get real* and deal with the emotional overlay as if it were one of your symptoms. Here are some stories from my clinical practice where a physical ailment was sourced and resolved by looking at the patients' emotional overlay.

Janet. Janet had been dealing with a pain in her right hip for several months. She had pursued nutritional supplements for arthritis, sought the help of a physical therapist for rehab of a past injury, and did yoga to address tight hip flexors. Being a nurse, she was knowledgeable about all of the probable anatomical and physiological causes. One day, after yoga class, her instructor suggested that she could be

....

11   Gareth Cook, "The Science of Healing Thoughts," in *Scientific American,* Jan, 19, 2016. www.scientificamerican.com/article/the-science-of-healing-thoughts/.

carrying anger in her hip and offered to have coffee with her to talk about it. Well, this suggestion made Janet furious! Who did he think he was anyway, suggesting her problem might be emotional? Was he trying to hit on her? Furthermore, her husband was constantly irritating her and there were some things she needed to tell him right away. Curiously, after giving expression to the litany of things that made her angry, Janet noticed that her hip no longer bothered her. Could it be that all of those irritating things were aggravating her hip? Could it be that she needed to give vent to everything that was a pain in the butt or making her angry before she could move forward in her life?

Carl. *Although Carl had no previous bronchial problems, he began to experience constriction in his chest and the symptoms of allergic asthma. He had been under medical care for several months when he was visited by his daughter on college vacation. When she left, he started to sob and sob, realizing that time had moved on and his precious little girl had grown to be a woman. His reaction totally surprised him, as he was philosophically at ease with her choices and proud of her independence. As Carl followed his sorrow, it led him on to grieving for his own youthfulness and the inevitable loss embodied in the passage of time. As the emotional flurry subsided, so did the pressure and congestion in his chest! It seemed that getting the emotional piece "off of his chest" was the key to breathing freely.*

Be honest. Being honest means looking at the whole picture and asking for help when you need it. If the emotional overlay is enmeshed and hard to separate, your physical healing might necessitate some emotional healing. A themed book or the counsel of a wise, mature friend or family member may be a good way to get some perspective, see what needs to be addressed, and get things moving. If your issues are more complicated, a professional therapist could be an essential addition to your healing team.

✿ Try This: The River of Life

A river metaphor is a helpful way to reassure your emotional body when your physical body is healing. Yes, you've left the Main Stream but you're still on the River of Life. You haven't been slammed, abandoned, sidelined, or isolated. You're just on a tributary of Rest and Restoration. Let yourself go with the flow and trust the River of Life—it will take you to your destination. Along the way, if you get sucked into eddies of fear, doubt, or despair, let go and surrender to the gentle tug of the current. If you come across a choppy piece of emotional turmoil, the best way to get through it is to go through it. If you encounter a rock (resistance) or sandbar (self-judgment), work on it until it dislodges. And if you discover you're carrying some emotional baggage, jettison it. As you float along, look for harbingers of hope and comfort along the way—a cloud formation, the appearance of a dove, wise words from a friend. Let the constancy of the river reassure your confidence and replenish your hope. Being on the River is about deep trust and deep faith. When you reach your destination, you'll know more about the being on the River of Life and who you are.

Change the story. Throughout time, every culture in the world has used universal themes, myths, and fables to impart vital wisdom and information for survival and healing. Use your imagination to construct a powerful story that contains important images for your healing. Just like the words and phrases shape your thoughts, the story you tell shapes how you think about sickness and injury. Listed below are some common overarching themes that correlate to proactive healing:

- Traveling into the underworld (forest/swamp/cave) to embrace the shadow (the hidden/the painful) in order to become a whole person.

- Breaking free from parents (the king/queen) in order to save the kingdom, find a solution, or forge new territory. All heroes and heroines have to leave home.

- Overcoming physical challenge and questioning established order in order to attain the prize.

- Being lost and meeting a wise elder/animal guide in order to find the way.

Any scenario with elements of challenge, exile, transformation, initiation, birthing, and/or dying can give you an overarching theme to reframe your story. To allow for perspective, see your story as a myth. Shift the setting to a different time and place; augment the circumstances to include a journey and a mega-theme; and give the major players powerful roles (seeker, king, warrior, sage, priest). As you concoct the storyline, don't be surprised if a victim or drill sergeant, stoic or dilettante, fool or scoundrel show up somewhere along the way. As you build the story, ask yourself: "What needs to be left behind? What needs to be accomplished? What tools or assistance would be helpful?" Even the shortest healing journey has challenges and setbacks that, when embraced, offer rewards of power and wisdom. Like others have discovered, you may be surprised how your healing myth unfolds. And, if the overarching theme wasn't apparent at the beginning of your story, rest assured that it will be at the end.

❀ Explore: Your Healing Journey

Get out your Body Wisdom journal, sit down, and gather in the details of your current situation. Engage your creative imagination and change the particulars of the story to design your own mythic journey. Use one of the overarching themes, assign the parts, and let your story tell itself. Where does your journey begin: at the edge of a forest, climbing a mountain, down the rabbit hole? Who is accompanying you? Be playful. What if your cast included animals or archetypal beings? Pick a couple randomly; you might be delighted by their uncanny perfection and symbolic message. What tools are you bringing with you—vision to see beyond the fog, a sword to pierce the veil, a compass to show the way? Who do you meet along the way? What gifts are you given? Look way out in the distance—can you see a clearing in the forest, light on the horizon, or a verdant distant shore? Bring it all together and write it down in your journal. Feel free to tap into the language and lore of fable and fairy tale to embellish the story. Look for recurring themes and archetypes. If you're inspired, illustrate it or include a poem.

Now stand back from what you've created. Does the myth you've concocted have something to tell you? Use the internet to research the symbolism of any object or living thing in your story. Isn't it interesting how your wise body slipped in just the right elements to give you some insight? Creating a healing myth gives you a way to see forces at play behind the scenes. Perhaps this journey was meant to be.

Fay. In her healing myth, Fay had the image of an abandoned castle represent her sick body and a battle-worn warrior standing at the edge of a forest surveying the scene. From this perspective, the castle was clearly unoccupied, crumbling, and overgrown. As the warrior watched, a little girl walked out of the castle and came toward him. He bent down to hear what she needed, and the little girl told him she was lonely and neglected and needed him to help get the castle back in order and full of life again. If the warrior could repair the ramparts (establish boundaries); clean the moat (get rid of old emotional baggage); stock the scullery (see to a healthy diet); and stoke the fires (replenish vitality), the child would have a safe home and the castle would be whole again. As the story proceeds, they run across an old groom who gives them the key to unlock the door to the inner chamber (heart). This healing myth helped Fay bring her little girl, her warrior, and her wise guide into a healing partnership to help her see the way to healing.

It changed the whole picture when Fay stepped away from her daily battle with chronic fatigue and let her healing myth tell her something. Somehow, her inner knowing designed the elements to reflect specific things she needed to do to get her castle-body in order. Now instead of feeling helpless and overwhelmed, she became a willing explorer on a symbolic journey.

Be Creative!

Healing from the inside means knowing how to find and use the extensive resources of your sentient body. These resources include both your cache of personal experience and your vast reservoir of ancestral wisdom. Whether you're dealing with a simple skinned knee, a stubborn virus, or a long-term healing crisis, get creative and step outside the box. Pivot slightly away from the rational, the linear, and tap into your imagination. It's time to leave the ordinary and set the stage for extraordinary healing.

Throughout the ages, healers have used the wisdom of the natural world to assist and augment the healing process. As Fay discovered earlier, when you tap into the dynamics of symbol and metaphor, you can look beyond, as well as within, for helpful allies and hidden assets for healing. If you're not familiar with visualizations, affirmations, and guided imagery, getting creative might feel strange and woo-woo at first. Remember that you have nothing to lose. It's time to break the hold of convention and activate your inner healer. Practice some of the following self-healing techniques and see what works for you. Listen to your wise body—it has the inside scoop. Trust your wise body—it's a faithful and honest guide. Show up 100 percent for your healing assignment and you can participate in miracles.

Self-Healing Strategies

Be with Nature

One way to heal from the inside is to get in touch with the outside. From a composition point of view, your body is intricately connected to the natural world—it's not so different from a rock or tree or star. And, just like everything in nature, your body has its basic needs, rhythms, and cycles. Studies have shown that when you're out of sync, your body is more likely to get sick or hurt. Living in a stimulus-driven, goal-oriented, techno-based society can undermine your natural balance. When was the last time you pulled away from the chaos and intensity to experience the unfettered simplicity of trees, birds, and fresh air? During my healing retreat programs, it was challenging for participants to sit for twenty minutes alone in the woods. Many people admitted they had never spent any time alone in nature. What about you?

Even if you don't have a health issue that you're aware of, connecting to the natural world is a healthy thing to do. Richard Louv, author of *The Nature Principle,* writes about the "nature deficit disorder" and makes a strong case for the healing powers of Vitamin N (nature). Not only does being in nature give you a transfusion of the essential elements for your natural balance but it also has something to teach you. Although being surrounded by wilderness is preferable, it's not the only place to get your Vitamin N. You can learn something about your body and recalibrate your wellness anytime you walk in a city park, sit in a garden, or look out the window. Just think of the elements of earth, water, fire, and air ... and you have nature.

✿ *Try This: Be with Nature*

Try one or more of the following ways to experience the healing power of nature. Notice how long it takes you to let go of your erratic pace and feel connected. Let your body slow down and settle in.

- Lie down and feel how gravity pulls you to the earth

- Get into water and feel your limbs float

- Let the warmth of the sun on your skin sink into your bones

- Close your eyes and feel the soft touch of air on your cheeks

- Sit with your back to a tree (or rock) and slow down to match its tempo

- Hear how your breath blends with the surrounding symphony
  of sounds

- Could you feel the tension soften as your experience expanded? Did
  you feel less isolated and more in tune afterward? Can you feel how
  your cells, bones, flesh, and breath are part of this natural world?

One of the first things you might notice when you go *au naturel* is the distraction and persistence of your busy mind. Rather than calculating your income for the week or recalling lyrics to a song, direct your attention to the sensual world around you. Be the curious observer and let nature tell the story. As you stay a little longer, you may begin to feel that you're a part of this place—if only for a short time. What if your pulsing and breathing body marked the passing of time like the movement of the breeze or the passing of the clouds? Go ahead, get creative and expand your healing horizons.

> *Marianne. When Marianne was diagnosed with a heart issue, her health team told her to reduce stress in her life. One morning while attending to her daily task of feeding the chickens on her ranch, she noticed how relaxed she felt. Sitting outside and watching the simple way the birds scratched and pecked made the complexities of her life recede in the background. For these few precious minutes, the pace of life slowed down and the center of the universe was the chicken yard. Connecting with nature helped Marianne's body and mind relax. Here, she felt the calm assurance that all was well in the world. Beginning her day with a dose of Vitamin N was just what her heart needed.*

> *Mark. A devastating virus affected Mark's balance for months. Although he was clearly getting better, his long recovery was only making him feel depressed, angry, and anxious rather than hopeful and encouraged. He couldn't return to his active life until he got his balance back. One day while walking on the beach, he felt the familiar*

angst close in on him. Rather than let his mind run wild with negative thoughts, Mark paused for a moment and turned his attention outward to the gentle, rhythmic ebb and flow of the water. As he stood there, he realized that his quest to find equilibrium was mental, as well as physical. And, just like the eternal movement of the tides, all was in perfect balance in his world. From then on, whenever he lost his balance, he remembered the lesson nature taught him at the beach. Connecting with the natural world helped him find patience with the healing process.

Being in nature helps you restore balance, feel connected, and reduce stress. Listening to nature can give you encouragement, answer a question, offer guidance, and precipitate insight. It can offer the poignant guidance and powerful information you need to grow and heal. For centuries, seers have used signs and symbols to bridge understanding between the physical and spiritual worlds. When you *get creative* and look at nature from a symbolic viewpoint, perhaps you've found a link to intuition.

❀ Try This: Find Your Charm

You've heard of people carrying a talisman or token (a rabbit's foot or St. Christopher's medal) for protection and fortitude. In the same way, you can get creative and find something significant to represent the presence of powerful forces and unseen allies on your healing journey. Anything you designate can be infused with intention for healing. Many Native American tribes use smoke from a bundle of dried cedar/sage to purify and carry a prayer to the Great Father/Mother. Ancient Sumerians wore amulets carved from stone for health and healing. Find your own special charm, give it significance, and keep it close by to remind you of the healing forces in nature. Here are some suggestions:

- A shell, stone, or piece of driftwood from the beach

- A photo of the Buddha, Mother Mary, or a rose in full bloom

- A piece of wood configured like a cross, a rock shaped like a heart, et cetera

- A metal charm of the yin/yang symbol or the goddess Gaia

Choose something that represents your need for purification, ageless wisdom, a benevolent guide, connection to spirit, or powerful allies. Use this symbol to help you anchor your faith in something bigger than your small self.

❀ *Try This: Listen to the Animals*

What if your deepest knowing wants to give you a clue or some guidance for your healing journey? One way to get your attention is by sending you a message from nature. The next time a random animal catches your attention (in real life, image, or dream), *get creative* and use your imagination. Listening to the animal kingdom means tapping in to the vast reservoir of cultural symbols, metaphors, and fables. Maybe an animal has already appeared. If not, look for one over the next day or two. After you give thanks to this animal for showing up, ask yourself:

- What does my animal typically symbolize in stories, fables, rhyme, or song?

- Do its mannerisms and attributes reveal something important at this time?

- Could its appearance be an asset, answer a question, or offer guidance?

To augment what you already know about this animal, search the internet for more ideas. Type in the name of the animal followed by the word *symbol*. Read a couple of different interpretations then come up with your own. Apply this to your present situation and see the significance. To decipher a message from the animal kingdom, you'll need to use your wide-angle lens, invite the full range of cultural intelligence, and look at the whole picture. Pay attention to any animal sighting; it could be an insightful message about your healing.

Here's how a couple of clients used the internet to *get creative* and listen to the animal kingdom:

Jacob. Jacob was in a high-powered job and his health was suffering from a Vitamin N deficiency. Feeling exhausted and depleted, he took a half day off and went into the woods behind his condo. As he walked, he noticed an owl sleeping in a sycamore tree. All he knew was that owls were considered wise. Later when he looked up owl symbol, *the internet offered him lots of ways to look at Owl. He found that this animal had accompanied the Greek goddess of wisdom, had extraordinary long-range vision, and was able to reveal unseen truths. Next, Jacob noted that the owl he saw was sleeping. It occurred to Jacob that Owl was urging him to get the rest he needed to have the vision and clarity to see how he might reset and reorder his priorities.*

Zev. *Zev dreamed about a mountain goat scaling high and difficult terrain. It certainly summed up how he felt in the third week of chemotherapy. When he checked the internet, Zev discovered that the goat meant both sure-footedness (in Chinese culture) and sacrifice (Old Testament). As he interpreted it, his goat was telling him that he could trust his body to find its way above the rocky slopes. In the meantime, if he let go of (sacrificed) his need for immediate results and took things step by step, the journey wouldn't seem so out of his control and scary.*

Spa@Home

By now, you know how important it is to unhook, de-stress, and give back to your body. Whenever you create a time and place to relax, replenish, and restore, your body literally soaks up the extra care and attention. This is especially important when you're sick or injured and need some healing. A good way to draw out physical and emotional toxins is the time-honored therapy of soaking in hot water. Combine any of the following elements to create your own spa@home:

The Setting. You can create a spa in your bathroom by lighting a candle and turning on soothing music. Dimmed lighting, bath salts, and fluffy towels help set the scene for relaxation and healing, in addition to whatever you think fosters an unhurried, calm atmosphere. Privacy is an important ingredient. You don't want to feel self-conscious if emotions happen to surface. Letting go physically and emotionally is an important part of healing.

The Treatment. Your simple spa@home menu includes an exfoliating scrub, detoxification soak, and self-massage. The first step begins before the bath as you dry brush or apply a scrub (commercial or olive oil/sea salt) to exfoliate and clean your pores. Then shower off and fill the bathtub with hot water, scented oils or Epsom salts and soak for ten or more minutes to relax and release toxins. (If you don't have a tub, stay a little longer in the shower and let the hot water cascade over your body and carry away all your tension and worry.) As you dry off, gently soothe and stimulate each part of your body. As a friend of mine used to say, "make sure you dry between each toe." Now give yourself a mini-massage with organic body oil or moisturizing cream.

The Rest. After your treatment, put on a robe and lie down someplace warm and comfy to let it all sink in. Focus your inner awareness on your healing as you let the gentle motion of your breath, the warmth, and self-care do their work. Think of your spa@home as a link to the ancient healing practices and miracles associated with water therapies around the world.

Energy Healing

Use your kinesthetic (spatial) sense to get creative and do some energy healing. Remember, this sense gives you information about internal/external space *and* energy fields. It is how you find your bedroom light switch in the dark, and how you feel the presence of a person or animal before you see them. This is also how you know if your body's relaxed or tense, open or closed. It's time to stretch a bit and use your spatial sense for energy healing.

❀ *Try This: Do-It-Yourself Energy Healing*

Lie down, close your eyes, make yourself comfortable, and imagine your body is a tube with energy flowing through it. Is the flow continuous, homogenous, and open? Or are there places that feel tight, stuck, thick, spiky, or closed? Can you make a connection between the healing you need to do and stuck energy flow? Is there an element of subtle muscular tension involved? If so, this is the time for some energy healing. To begin, bring your awareness to the specific epicenter of the problem and describe the feeling.

- Is the area denser/thicker as if the cells were packed together?

- Does it feel distant or numb?

- Is your awareness going around instead of through this place?

- Does the temperature feel colder or hotter?

- Is it hyperalert and/or isolated in pain or discomfort?

All the above are indicators of a blocked energy flow. If your energy is blocked, sapped or trapped, it's not available for healing. Rather than go into the reasons why this may be so, just do some energy healing and get it going again. Use your imagination to soften, expand, or free it up and open the flow. Let the palms of your hands emanate warmth, cooling, serenity, light, or healing colors. Use your fingertips to brush away discord, old memories, or emotional debris. Picture the flow opening so energy can move through, soothing and balancing. And, as the area begins to open up, imagine the flow delivering everything your body needs for healing. It really doesn't matter whether you actually *feel* the energy or simply use the image to construct a powerful visualization.

Research has shown that getting things moving through yoga and tai chi improves circulation, mood, and overall vitality.[12] Whether you're on a healing journey or not, checking your energy flow and doing some energy healing periodically is good for your health.

Visualizations and Affirmations

Visualizations, affirmations, and prayer are ways to get your mind and emotions aligned for healing. Research shows that aligning belief with your healing intention is a good way to reduce surgical complications and speed up recovery.[13] Because a health crisis asks you to trust your smart body just when your confidence feels the lowest, being conscious of the message you're sending is doubly important. If your personal sound bites, self-talk, and Emotional Intake interview have revealed some negatives, get creative and design specific positive pictures/words for your situation. For instance, if your hurt back includes the feeling that no one "has your back," your positive visualization might be imagining that you're "leaning back" in the supportive embrace of loved ones, professional helpers, and unseen helpers. Your affirmation could be "I have all the *backing* I need."

....

12   Catherine Woodyard, "Exploring the Therapeutic Effects of Yoga and Its Ability to Increase Quality of Life," in *International Journal of Yoga,* Jul–Dec 2011. ncbi.nlm.nih.gov/pmc/articles /PMC193654/.

13   Chittaranjan Andrade, "Prayer and Healing: A Medical and Scientific Perspective on Randomized Controlled Trials," in *Indian Journal of Psychiatry,* Oct–Dec 2009. www.ncbi.nlm .nih.gov/pmc/articles/PMC2802370/.

Here are some visualizations that affirm healing:

- Picture your body sitting in a field of golden light. Each inhale brings a great healing light into your body. All refuse and negativity is released in each exhale. With each cycle of breathing, you're inhaling the essence of radiant wellness and exhaling the substance of sickness or injury. In this process, each and every cell is infused with space, ease, and vitality. Each and every cell is cleared of tension, pain, and dis-ease.

- Let your hands (or your attention) connect with the place that needs healing. Notice how this place might feel slightly different from the surrounding area. Maybe there is a certain density, intensity, and/or pain. See this discomfort as crowded cells and compressed tissue. Bring your awareness into the epicenter and let it get really, really big. Feel the density (discomfort, intensity, pain) dissipate. Keep expanding and letting go until there is only space and no matter. This visualization is excellent for anchoring healing intention and alleviating pain.

Here are some generic affirmations to consider for healing:

- "Healing happens from the inside out."
- "My body was designed to heal."
- "I am in the center of a vortex of healing light."
- "Each day, in every way, I am getting better and better."
- "My feet are guided and grounded on a steady path to healing."

Your mind will be comforted to know that your creative affirmations and visualizations can actually work. You don't need a double-blind study to validate these body-smart techniques. Just find a positive statement and/or image and be with it once a day. Your body will get the message.

🌸 *Try This: An Attitude of Gratitude*

It's simply impossible to be grateful and negative at the same time. Changing your personal statement from resentment or blame to appreciation and thanks could be a significant step toward healing. As an ongoing practice, it'll also change your life's dynamic. A key factor in all successful recovery programs is cultivating an attitude of gratitude. Instead of circulating the same old stinkin' thinkin', try starting your day with:

- "I am grateful for the vitality that moves through every cell and atom of my body. I acknowledge all of the external and internal sources of help that are aligned with my healing."

- "I am thankful for all of the ways that my body serves me, cares for me, protects me, and is always there for me. I acknowledge my sacred stewardship for this vessel and am open to the help I need in order to heal."

If these phrases don't suit you, use your imagination and design your own. Even if you don't feel particularly grateful at the moment, throw together some positive words, try it out for a couple of days, and feel what happens. As you discovered in this chapter, being positive has an uplifting effect on your physiology even if it's rote or performed.

Create Ceremony

Ritual and ceremony bring a sacred element to your healing journey. The truth is, total healing entails more than rebalancing, repairing, and recovering. Your body might be sick or injured, but your whole being might also be out of balance and in need of healing. When your healing journey includes and reaffirms a connection to a greater whole (family, community, nature, and the mystery of life), it's more than physical—it's spiritual.

Including a spiritual dimension on the healing journey is both practical and functional. Medical research has shown that prayer even by strangers can reduce postsurgical complications and speed recovery time. In addition, there are innumerable anecdotal stories linking prayerful intentions and positive results. Placebo or not, creating a ceremony (vision circle, prayer circle, or whatever title feels comfortable), helps you validate your process, ask for what you need, and feel supported. It can also give your loved ones a way to feel included and helpful.

Design your healing ceremony to suit your circumstances. Many people feel awkward asking for help, being the center of attention, or participating in unfamiliar rituals. For this reason, you'll want to keep your ceremony simple and personal. See it as a gathering in of loved ones and an artistic way of asking for help. Be creative and get personal. Using your specific situation and aesthetics to construct a ceremony can make the experience easy, enjoyable, and effective.

Remember that sweet and simple are best and don't forget to ask for what you need. It can be effective to empower the moments at the beginning or ending with prayers, poetry, music, or a few moments of silence. You can stand in the middle and receive blessing; you can hold hands or sing a song together. The ceremony is about you and whatever works for you.

If you don't feel up to the task, ask for help. After all, the idea is about recruiting all your resources—seen and unseen. Creating ceremony isn't a small-self endeavor; it's about your big self and an ageless community/tribal tradition. Participating in a healing ceremony is a way to confirm interconnectedness and meaning in life. It's centering to set the intention as well as the sacred space. It's calming to choose the candles, flowers, beautiful fabrics, and symbolic objects. It's empowering to design the program with positive messages and images. And, it's reassuring to come together and hold a collective intention. Creating ceremony may be the most powerful thing you do on your healing journey.

Bess. *Bess was scheduled for surgery and wanted to design a ceremony for a circle of loved ones to ask them to hold good thoughts for her and her medical team. Beforehand, she set the sacred space by cleaning her home, putting chairs in a circle, and placing meaningful objects (candles and a picture of a holy teacher) in the center. She also designed the format of her ceremony beginning with a piece of favorite music and words of welcome and gratitude. When the day arrived and after bringing everyone up to date on her health situation, Bess passed a basket full of beach stones around the room and asked each person to take a stone and give an offering in the form of a prayer, blessing, or good wishes. Bess asked her guests to hold their stones to represent their good thoughts and wishes as a way to help her heal. When the big day arrived, Bess felt comfort and confidence knowing that her healing circle and their love were with her.*

Liam. *Struggling with a long-term illness, Liam felt totally depleted and needed an energy infusion. A friend offered to organize a small and heartfelt event to help out. Because their community was eclectic spiritually, they settled on a potluck format. Everyone would bring food for the potluck and something to put in Liam's freezer. People were also given a brief update of Liam's condition and needs, and they were encouraged to think about how they might help. When the day came, a spontaneous ceremony casually unfolded in Liam's living room. It included a reiteration of help he needed and a heartfelt appreciation for everyone present. There was a basket by the door where people could put little notes of personal encouragement, offers of support (including taxi service, house cleaning, back rubs, and shopping), and financial contributions. In the end, the ceremony worked for everyone. The love, care, and good will gave Liam the infusion he needed and the sentiment of the event brought a little healing into everyone's life.*

There's a pivotal moment when a healing journey crests the uphill climb and recovery is on the horizon. As you return to the fullness of health, give yourself time to reflect on where you've been and what you've learned. When you began your journey, you accepted your challenge and made it personal. You put yourself in the driver's seat and listened to inner knowing as you sought help and followed protocols for getting well. Along the way, your smart body was there to course-correct, add insight, and follow through. Over and over again, as you took each turn, hope was rekindled and meaning discovered. You even went a step beyond and did some personal exploring to help your body heal and stay healthy. Everything you've experienced has helped your mind move beyond fear, denial, blame, or magical thinking to a deeper trust in the wisdom of your body. Through it all, you were not alone. In times of confusion there was faith. In times of need there was help. In times of doubt there was synchronicity. The challenges and the blessings have forged a new understanding of who you are and the life you live.

Even when healing doesn't mean curing, if you show up and embrace the journey, your wisdom will grow, and so will your spirit. Take a moment now to acknowledge what you've learned. Ask yourself these questions and write the answers in your Body Wisdom journal:

- What have I discovered about myself/the experience of being alive?

- How has this healing journey changed the way I feel about my body?

- What have I learned about the body-mind connection?

- Did moments of synchronicity confirm the interconnectedness of people/circumstance?

- Did my time out give me a chance to re-evaluate relationships, choices, and priorities?

- What kind of emotional clearing transpired along the way?

- How am I different today?

- How did my wise body help me through?

Any healing journey has the potential to change your relationship with your body and give you a deeper understanding of the mystery of life. In a certain sense, no matter what your circumstances or where you're standing on the path to wellness, the healing never stops. Your body is a work in progress. And, the health of your body, mind, and spirit are interconnected and dynamic. Healing is about being whole. Now it's time to take the wisdom you've accrued and venture forth and explore your emotional, intuitive, and spiritual body.

Six
The Emotional Body

Like a filter applied over perception, the experience of your emotional body colors your thoughts, relationships, decisions, opinions, communication, and everything you think and do. Emotion influences the way you see the world and the way the world sees you. This gets reaffirmed over and over again in your personal life. If there is emotional turmoil, your focus is fuzzy and your mind is muddled. If you're elated, confused, excited, or frustrated, it affects your viewpoint, stamina, and physical strength. When you feel stressed out, your tolerance and resilience are diminished. When you're calm and centered, it's easier to find the words to express your ideas. This chapter will help you connect all the dots so you can understand, feel comfortable, and know how to take care of your emotional body.

Meet Your Emotional Body

Of course you know how emotion feels in your body. Sadness collapses, puckers, and floods. Fear clutches, dampens, and trembles. Anger tightens, shakes, and spikes. Joy pulses, sways, and soars. Sadness, fear, anger, and joy are examples of how your emotional body interacts with the ups and downs of life. It may surprise you to know that these same responses are simply a part of the emotional design of all humans whether in the jungles of New Guinea, a high-rise in Beijing, or a monastery in upstate New York.[14] It's a stimulus-response kind of reaction. When your emotional response is inappropriate or holds on for days or even years, the design has malfunctioned. One way or the other, when emotion comes along and doesn't go along, it takes root and can become hardwired. When that happens, the emotional impression becomes your personal expression. Chances are you can find some emotional history set in your own muscle tension.

✤ Try This: Wearing Emotions

You can feel the impression of your emotional history in your body. Even if you're not feeling any overt emotion right now, old events and unresolved relationships may still be informing the shape and intensity of your physical tension. To explore this possibility, take a few moments to sit quietly, close your eyes, and feel what's going on. As you let go of the top layer of tension, what do you find underneath? Can you feel the shape of a familiar expression still set in your face? Do some muscle groups continue to hold on, up, or in? If there's no physical reason for your clenching jaw, squeezing buttocks, pinching forehead, pushing tongue, or bunching stomach, there may be an emotional reason. Tighten in a little more and ask your body-mind, "What emotion lives here?" It could be anger, fear, sorrow, anticipation, disgust, pride, or something else, but don't try to figure it out at this point. Just listen to the first thing that pops into your mind. When you match up the physical feeling with the emotional feeling, your history shows up to say, "Here I am." In order to let go of this emotional tension, you'll need to listen to your emotional body.

> *Angela. Angela encountered her emotional body on the massage table. She noticed that as the rest of her body started to relax, her hands curled into tight fists. Her therapist suggested that maybe her emotional body had something to say. Her very first thought was that she was handling too much with too little help. This imbalance was a familiar scenario, and her emotional body was holding on to some anger and resentment as a result. When she opened her hands to let go and receive the help she*

---

14   Wellcome Trust, "Everybody laughs, everybody cries: Researchers identify universal emotions," in *Science Daily*, Jan 26, 2010. www.sciencedaily.com/releases/2010/01 /100125173234.htm.

needed, the gesture brought on hot tears. Once Angela's emotional body let go, her physical body could open to receive the massage.

❁ *Try This: What Can Tension Tell You?*

What if your unconscious, physical tension is informed by some emotional history? To explore this possibility, return to what you discovered in the emotional tension exercise above and figure it out. Let your skeptical mind step aside and your curious mind step forward. Give your imagination free reign as you play a game of cause and effect. When you ask your body what's really going on, it's surprising how literal your body can be. Here are some emotional body connections that make sense:

- If your jaw is clamped shut, you might be afraid to speak your truth.

- If you have a pain in the backside, you could be sitting on your anger.

- If your forehead is pinched, you might be worried about what's ahead.

- If your chest is tight, it might be sheltering some heartache.

- If you have a tense stomach, maybe there's something that's hard to stomach.

In order to find the underlying cause, you may need to suspend a belief that your shoulders are tight simply because that's where you carry tension, your lower back is stiff because of a weakness or injury, or your brow is furrowed because your father furrowed his brow. It's helpful to be creative, playful, and bold when you set out to hear what your emotional body has to say. Listen for the enigmatic, symbolic message.

Emotional Posture

Your tension and postural patterns confirm the principle that form follows function, and we're not just talking about use and workload; it's also about drama and trauma. When you have unresolved emotional issues, they inform your tension and imprint your posture. Many body-oriented therapists and structural body workers acknowledge the formative relationship between emotion and posture. Knowing this, they work through the body to address the underlying emotional issues.[15] The rationale is simple—when you hold on to the issues, your body holds on (bracing, protecting, deflecting, and managing). When you can get the body to let go, the underlying emotions surface and let go as well. When you aren't saddled with emotional backlog, your emotional posture doesn't need to be shaped by the past. The result is greater comfort, less pain, better posture, and more flexibility.[16]

✿ Try This: What's Your Posture Holding?

Many people don't know what to do with their emotions, and end up storing them in their body. Once there, the emotional tension begins to shape their physical tension. If your emotional history has informed (think: "in-formed") your posture, it may be time to feel it and heal it. Here are some correlations you might find:

- Sunken chest holding on to disappointment

- Clamped jaw squaring off for a fight

- Scrunched neck shrinking from fear

- Raised shoulders bracing against a threat

- Tucked tummy holding some anger

- Squeezed buttocks holding back pleasure

Of course, your sunken chest might be about fear or your raised shoulders about something else. Listen to your body; it knows what your emotional posture is holding. As you become more body-conscious, it's pretty clear how a favorite holding pattern dovetails with a specific emotional construct. Long established emotional postures are often

....

15 Nadia Bianchi-Berthouze, Paul Cairns, Anna Cox, Charlene Jennet, and Whan Woong Kim, "On Posture as a Modality for Expression and Recognizing Emotions," uclic.ucl.ac.uk /publications/237582.

16 Kristin V. Brown, "How Posture Influences Mood, Energy, and Thoughts," in *SFGate*, September 3, 2013. sfgate.com/health/article/How-postrue-influences-mood-energy -thoughts-4784543.php.

deeply entrenched in habit and personality. Although they may feel like normal, they're restrictive, effortful, and hold you back. Read on to learn how your body-oriented awareness can help you extricate your posture from its emotional history.

Body Armor

Your emotional posture is your way of dealing with and adapting to the ups and downs of your personal history. It's also a significant part of your defense system. Your emotional body uses muscle tension to keep feelings in and harm out. You can feel this happen even when something small and incidental touches an emotion and your muscles tighten slightly. This is how it works: if you want to protect yourself, your body will bulk up; if you want to avoid all feeling, your body will become numb; if you want to brace yourself against criticism, your body will tighten up. This is called *body armor*.

> **Steve.** *Steve looked at the pictures from his thirtieth birthday party and was dismayed to see his old postural habits in full display. Although he thought he was enjoying the festivities, it didn't look like it. His emotional posture looked deflated, beleaguered, and distracted. By exaggerating the familiar slump, he could feel the impression of his emotional history—the youngster who felt awkward and the teenager who felt judged. Years ago this posture may have provided a place of refuge but in the present it was holding him hostage to the past, restricting his spontaneity and authenticity.*

> **Julia.** *Julia's life had dealt her the perfect storm of stress. She was divorcing her husband, had just sold their home, and needed to move. Then, her father died and the city cited the estate for code violations on one of his commercial properties. No wonder her body was in defense mode and she was unable to relax. When Julia sought much-needed rest at night, she was thwarted by the revved up tension in her emotional body. Her shoulders and neck were on guard as if she had her hackles up. One night Julia just let herself quake and cry it out. When she was finished, her emotional tension had diffused. Taking off her emotional body armor made it possible to surrender to the physical fatigue and go to sleep. After all, she could always armor up again in the morning if necessary.*

Anytime your body or psyche needs protection, your emotional body armors up for protection, which can be helpful in the moment. But like Steve and Julia, if you put the armor on and leave it on, it ends up getting in the way. Instead of deflecting harm, it distracts, disorients, inhibits, and isolates. Tragically, when your muscles are locked down in defense mode every day, your posture eventually takes on a personality of its own. Your armored stance limits perception, restricts movement, consumes energy, and keeps you on guard whether you need it or not. When any tension in your body simply feels normal, intractable, or hardwired, it has become a part of your emotional posture. Body-oriented therapists believe that addressing emotional posture is a key to healing the mind and body. In their work, they often see a slumped posture reclaim its full height slowly but surely when the hold of grief is broken. Or, observe a body begin to move freely and gracefully when the stranglehold of anger is released.

Emotional Expression

The muscles of your face have an emotional range. Take a moment to feel the versatility as you shift your expression from eager to skeptical to confused to bored and unreceptive. When these expressions are linked with real stimuli, they move across your face as situations come and go. Yet just like your posture, your face can be a repository for emotions to hang out and hang on. Observe the muscles of your face when you're solving a tough problem, sitting in a traffic jam, or concentrating on a new idea in this book. As you figure, stew, or ruminate, can you feel your muscles pull into expressions of scrutiny, irritation, or concentration? Your emotional expression is perfectly suited to the moment. If it lingers and becomes habitual, however, your emotional expression is locked in and you lose a valuable communication tool. Remember that even a smile can get frozen in place and become a holding pattern.

Researchers have identified over twenty distinct facial expressions.[17] However, most people use only two or three. Check out the faces of friends or public figures that haven't undergone cosmetic procedures. Imagine what muscles are contracting and what message

....

17   Bahar Gholipour, "Happily Surprised! People Use More Facial Expressions Than Thought,"
      Live Science-Health, March 31, 2014, www.livescience.com/44494-human-facial-expressions
      -compound-emotions.html.

they communicate. Why do some of these faces have pinched foreheads (eyes or lips)? Why do some look objectively happy and peaceful and others look angry, sad, or worried? Could some of these expressions reflect a default emotion rather than a legitimate response to the moment? Let the muscles of your own face squeeze and pull to mimic these expressions. What emotions do they feel like? Your facial expression is a powerful communicator. What if it tells the same old story over and over again? Chances are that the message you are sending is neither accurate nor spontaneous.

❀ *Try This: Your Dominant Expression*

Have you ever noticed how a baby's face is constantly changing, reflecting the emotional tenor of each moment? In contrast, by the time you become an adult, your emotional expression may have only a couple of options. Sadly, although you have the muscular ability, your emotional expression is stuck—the older you are, the more stuck it gets. To identify your dominant emotional expression, stand in front of a mirror and close your eyes. Feel the residual tension in your face. Can you feel your muscles tug and pull your lips, cheeks, forehead, and so forth into a certain shape? Now squeeze them a little more to exaggerate. Open your eyes. Can you see an emotional tone or message in your expression? Because this is your face, after all, stay curious rather than critical. Simply assess the expression and its tone. Does the message align with a dominant theme or familiar feeling in your life? For example:

- Does your forehead scrunch with worry, concern, or anticipation?

- Does your mouth pull down with disgust, anger, or disappointment?

- Do your eyes squint with sorrow, fear, or confusion?

- Does your brow furrow with angst, judgment, or rage?

- Or, does your expression have other things to communicate?

How you face and stand in the world tells a lot about you and your emotional body, and the message is louder than your words. Think about it—your postural and facial expressions are powerful nonverbal communicators. Your emotional body is sending messages every minute about who you are and what you feel. At the same time, consciously or unconsciously, you're getting cues and making assumptions based on the expression of every person you encounter. When you understand how your emotional body functions, you can begin to unravel the tension at the source and make sure your expression matches your intention.

Understanding the Emotional Body

To your controlling and analytical mind, living in an emotional body can feel untidy, unpredictable, and uncomfortable. Perhaps in part this is why your mind tries so hard to deny, distract, and circumvent your feelings. However, having emotions is part of the package, and when emotions surface, they need to move. If they don't, you end up with more and more buried feelings that consume more and more energy and space. Understanding the physical properties and basic nature of your emotional body is a straightforward way to clean up the backlog and establish good emotional hygiene.

Let's begin with the obvious. Emotions are triggered by circumstance and memory. Although your mind identifies and describes the experience, feeling and expressing are the purview of your body. Fear, grief, joy, anxiety, frustration, anticipation, disgust, compassion, and love each have a unique physical profile. Consider the full cycle of sadness: your chest collapses, cheeks pucker, throat tightens, eyes tear up, breath gets uneven, and a sob comes out. Consider the full cycle of anger: your jaw tightens, stomach tenses, adrenalin flutters, fists clench, and volume increases. Even a random thought or a story from a book, movie, or a friend's sharing can evoke a split second of sorrow, irritation, or glee that registers in your emotional body. This is why we feel touched by emotions. Yet, if your emotional body feels it and doesn't express it, where did it go?

✿ Try This: Emotion Is Moving Energy

In physics equations, the letter e represents energy. Considering "e-motion" as energy in motion is a good way to conceptualize how feelings travel through your body. For instance, fear's journey might be a flow of adrenalin with a vibration of trembling and humming. Joy's pathway might include a wave of euphoria, expansive gestures, and a percussive shout. The next time you're at the movies, immersed in a novel, or listening to the news and something triggers your feelings, see if you can sense the energy. Notice how it flows differently as fear, grief, pride, and hope. Once you identify the e (energy) part of the equation, feel the movement part. If you're in a private place, see if you can find a sound and gesture to enhance the momentum. Let the e-motion flow through and out of your body. It's as simple as that.

You can feel the unique muscular signature and energy current when an emotion is brewing. Anger feels different than grief; joy feels different than worry. But in life, you know that anger doesn't last very long and joy is fleeting. A healthy emotional body is always shifting and changing. Emotions come up, move through, and move on. But if they don't move on and get stuck, your body is left holding the bag. If you're all wrapped up in the tensions and postures of old events and feelings, you lose perspective, resiliency, choice, and finesse. Tending to emotional hygiene and healing will help you show up today with clarity and focus.

Emotional Hygiene

To be alive is to have feelings—mild or intense, coming or going. Your emotional life has a very physical presence in the way your feelings register, move, and express through your body. Like food consumed, digested, and expelled, your e-motions need to move on through. A stuck or sluggish emotional body is uncomfortable, unnatural, and unhealthy. The health of your body *and* psyche depends on good emotional hygiene, something just as important as eating well and getting enough sleep.

✿ Explore: Emotion Is Moving Energy

Pay attention to how your emotions imprint your body for a couple of days. Don't analyze why you're feeling something, just observe how and where they register in your body. A good time to do this is after an emotional event or first thing in the morning. At these times, your feelings are close to the surface. Here are some things you might want to note and record in your Body Wisdom journal:

- Sensual impressions (texture, color, density)

- Where you feel supercharged, numb, or blocked

- Muscle groups that are engaged, clenched, braced, or pinched

- Mood sensations such as jumpiness, irritability, or restlessness

- Connection between a physical sensation and how you feel

As you follow the daily ebb and flow of e-motion in your physical body, you might notice that certain tensions and feelings seem to repeat over and over. These could be indicators of something deeply rooted in your personal history. If so, they will need a bit of processing and healing before they move on. Once you understand how it works, good emotional hygiene is simple.

As you tuned in to the physicality of your e-motions, you recorded a moment in time. Hopefully you also noticed the energy's natural impetus to move and move on. Healthy hygiene means motility rather than stagnation. Like other flowing things in your body such as sweat, blood, and lymph, when e-motions come along and don't keep going along, they clog up the works. You can actually feel it, too. Some distinctive indicators of blocked emotional energy are:

- Heaviness around the eyes
- An inability to be quiet and sit still
- Churning in the gut
- Pervasive irritability and/or fatigue
- Any numbness, tightness, or pain
- Difficulty staying present or focusing
- Digestive or sleep disorders

When you become aware of blocked emotional energy, it's helpful to remember that like any holding pattern, the emotional tension in your body is not set in stone. When you emphasize physical expression and clearing rather than cognitive content and understanding, it's like going through the back door where you don't have to wrestle with your wily mind. The goal is simply a healthy and well-functioning emotional body.

Five Steps for Emotional Hygiene

Emotional hygiene means having feelings, not suppressing them. Because emoting on the spot is often counterproductive, it's important to establish a regular practice to deal with both current and restimulated feelings. Seeing this as just another avenue for self-care helps facilitate and demystify the process. So whenever you encounter a provocative situation or feel a buildup of emotional tension, follow these steps: set it up, get into it, experience it, be done with it, and let it go.

1. Set It Up

The beginning and end of the day are good times to check in and attend to your emotional hygiene. A daily practice ensures that you stay current with your feelings and avoid a slow buildup of emotional tension. Checking in regularly gives you a good baseline to know whether or not you have some "emotional flossing" to do. Because this is personal and private, you'll want to choose a time and place where you can feel safe and uninhibited. If other people (or even pets) are in close proximity, be sure to let them know that you might be moving some emotional energy and there's no need to be alarmed. If this isn't comfortable for them, it won't be comfortable for you.

2. Get Into It

Scan your body and feel where the emotional charge and tension are occupying space. Find some words to describe the sensations and how they influence your comfort and movement. Maybe the emotional energy feels sluggish or trapped, gray or red, pulsating or dull, loud or silent. Maybe your body feels jittery or stiff, tired or pumped, weak or hesitant. This is not about figuring it out or going into the whys and wherefores. It's about feeling the physical qualities of location and sensation.

3. Experience It

Once you feel it in your body, sink into the experience of it. Ask yourself: "What does this feeling look and sound like?" Find the precise movements and sounds and let your body express the feelings. Being authentic is both the practice and the purpose; there is no performing here. Once you get your e-motions moving, check your body again for clarity, asking: "Is this all of it or has another place/feeling surfaced that needs its own expression?" Remember that anger can lead to sorrow; fear can lead to laughter; frustration can lead to joy. (Yes, even joy gets stuck.)

4. Be Done with It

Keep expressing your feelings (gestures and sounds) until your e-motions are spent. Reassure your mind that the sobbing, howling, and trembling won't go on and on forever (simple authentic emoting often takes between one and five minutes). Check in and notice how your body feels once you're done with it. Once the channels are clear, the calm and focus establish a reference point for neutral in your emotional body.

5. Let It Go

This final step is absolutely essential. Before you return to your active, engaged life, make sure you let it all go. Release any lingering content, images, and intensity that triggered and/or accompanied your emotional session. One way to think of it is that emotions are messy so you need to clean up afterward. It's kind of like taking a shower after a heavy workout to wash off the sweat. Letting it go means directing all images and memories out of your energy field.

Even if you can't feel it, take a moment and imagine the energy moving like sound waves out and away from your body. Try using something symbolic (lighting candles, smudging with dried herbs, taking a purifying bath) to help you let it all go.

Break the Code of Silence

Following the five-step protocol may be the first time you've actually encouraged your body to be both the context and the conduit for your emotions. Don't be surprised if you encounter some resistance and backtalk when you first start. And certainly don't be discouraged if you find it challenging to express yourself freely. After all, you're bucking up against years of avoidance and suppression backed by a pretty powerful cultural demand to keep a lid on it. Here are a couple of ways to overcome the code of silence and get it moving:

The Alchemy of Release

Emotions have different profiles. Some are naturally jerky, some kinetic, some slow, some pulsing, some punching, and some shaking. Don't focus on naming the emotion. Just find the movement that matches the feeling. Once you get the movement, add the soundtrack, keeping in mind that you don't have to be loud to be authentic. When you get the alchemy of release right, you'll know it. The heaviness of your e-motional disturbance will transform into the lightness of deep peace and contentment. I've told many people that when you find the precise sound and gesture to free your emotions, you can turn lead into gold.

Scoop It Up and Throw It Away

Emotions always have an epicenter. When various feelings are triggered, not only do they have a distinct feeling, they show up in your body in different places. For instance, anger will sometimes tighten the thighs, fear will grip the pelvis, and sorrow will tighten the chest. Once you identify the location of the emotional disturbance, grab—or scoop, sweep, or brush—the contents and fling them into the air and off to the horizon. Scoop up the disturbance as if it were solid content and throw it away. No matter your method for disposal, the message here is clear: you are *not* your emotions. Your emotions are simply energy that needs to move … and you're moving it. Imagine that each time you scoop and throw, your stockpile is substantively decreased. Although this seems pretty simplistic, you'll feel the results.

Hear the Tone

Put your hand on any place on your body that's tense, numb, overcharged, or painful and give it your full attention. Keeping your attention centered, use your voice and generate a tone from this place. Listen to and hear the emotional tenor of this sound. What message does it convey? What if you increased the volume a bit and exaggerated the sound to *be* the emotion? Try it out and feel what movement might accompany the sound. Toning and moving without a story is a good way to circumvent the busy, bossy mind and give your feeling body a voice. Later you can ask, "What's going on?" and "What do I need?"

Scared Bunny, Angry Bear

If expressing your feelings strikes you as awkward or threatening, it may be hard to find even the softest sound or slightest movement in your emotional body. Let's face it—there are rewards for being nice-nice and punishments for letting emotions fly built within our culture. Often, men have a hard time with fear; women have a hard time with anger. Because the animal kingdom doesn't have the same restriction, it might be able to help you find and express your emotions. A good way to connect with your feelings and get them moving is to mimic a scared bunny or an angry bear. How do you know the bunny is scared? It squeaks a little and shakes like it is cold. How do you know a bear is angry? It careens around erratically, swatting and snarling. See if you can find the soundtrack and choreograph the dance moves for your animal—exasperated bumble bee, joyful whale, disgusted lion, grieving baboon, loving puppy. Calling on the animal kingdom is a good way to circumvent your verbal mind and find your emotional body's authentic expression.

If you commit yourself to having good e-hygiene, you can count on some good results. In a very short time, the confining need to be on top of everything and keep it all together will give way and afford you the space to explore, find creative solutions, and be spontaneous. In addition, when you live in an aware body and keep it all moving, your relationship with your emotional self will change. No longer is it the unruly wild-card that can throw you off and ruin everything. No longer is it something you need to silence, hide, regret, or push away; instead, it's just another part of being alive. As you become more familiar with how they work, your e-motions won't seem so mysterious or foreign any more. Do you notice how feelings come and go like weather? Do you have a sense of what being emotionally neutral feels like? Has the turmoil, chaos, and drama of your everyday life diminished? Understanding your emotional body changes your idea of what it means to be a sentient human being. As you will discover in the next chapter, your emotional body plays a big role in communicating the subtle messages that underlie successful relationships and good instincts.

Sophia. Sophia had established a good practice of emotional hygiene. For the most part, she traveled through life on an even keel and, when necessary, did the five steps process. When her husband got sick, she realized that some of her emotional calm was actually sourced in his reliable strength. Without her rock, old fears surfaced. Just when she needed to be steady and strong, she felt uncertain and weak. She noticed that everything seemed to be centered in her churning, quaking gut. Her emotional body was shouting at her and hard to overlook. Knowing how to proceed, Sophia set up some private time to get the e-motion moving. She told her husband and kids not

to be alarmed if they heard loud strange sounds, that it was just some energy she was
releasing. Once she got it set up, Sophia tuned in to the upset in her body and searched
for the sounds and gestures that connected with what she felt. As she rocked back and
forth, cradling her tummy, her exhale expressed a visceral, vibrating sound. As the
e-motion moved up and out of her body, she could feel the discomfort dissipate and
a calm settle in. Not only did this clear her emotions but it gave her the strength and
clarity to handle the demands and uncertainties of the next day.

Carlo. Carlo was in the throes of a painful divorce. His whole life was in upheaval,
and all the issues he'd tucked away were flooding to the foreground. He needed to
be able to focus on getting his life put together, but he was distracted, confused, and
stuck. At first when I suggested that he clear his emotional body every morning in
order to clear his mind, he thought it would be one more distraction that would only
bring up too much old baggage. Like many people, Carlo assumed that once you
open the floodgates, there's no closing them. Learning the five steps process gave him
a way to deal with his feelings in the simplicity of his body. On the days he did his
five steps, Carlo noticed his mind was focused and clear. As an added bonus, he felt
hopeful about the future. It was clear for Carlo that getting his emotions moving was
essential to helping him move on.

Whenever your emotions surface, make sure to set aside some time for e-hygiene. Like Sophia and Carlo discovered, you can expect to find relief and clarity following an emotional catharsis. When the storm clears, the fog will lift.

Your daily commitment to emotional hygiene comes in handy anytime you feel overwhelmed, blindsided, or unable to cope. The more intense the situation, the more you need to trust the physical process. Your wise body can help you be your best in the worst times if you give yourself the time and space to connect with your e-motions and keep them flowing. Of course, it's also good to remember your de-stressing strategies from chapter 6 so you can stay grounded and centered until the upheaval and intensity subside.

Cut yourself some slack if once in a while you don't have a chance to set it up and do the five steps. Sometimes stuff happens and the circumstances of life hit you like a tsunami. Anytime you encounter a situation that evokes core grief or fear, it may feel impossible to do anything but emote on the spot—know this is appropriate. Sorrow floods forth at a memorial; fear rattles after a trauma. This is your emotional body being healthy and healing. As a social being, you've held the space for others to dissolve or collapse emotionally, so don't apologize or shame yourself for taking your turn.

Finding Neutral

Good e-hygiene doesn't come naturally. You'll definitely need to practice in order to become good at it. The theory is easy to grasp, however, because you know that your emotional work begins and ends in your body. Simplistically, when emotional energy is activated, it takes shape in your body (your tension, posture, and demeanor) and needs to be expressed by sound or gesture *through* your body so that you can move on. Even though you may feel mentally and philosophically at peace, if your feelings are suppressed, your emotional body is unsettled. If your feelings have been processed and moved along, you can rest in neutral. Being in neutral means that your emotional expression is no longer impressed by the issue or event. There's no clamped jaw, fluttery belly, or foggy head. Even if your mind goes there again, your body doesn't.

Being in neutral is the baseline for accurate perception, uncluttered focus, inspired creativity, uncomplicated communication, and peaceful contemplation. Being in neutral is a wonderful place to hang out. As a reference point, it generates a kind of calm/certainty that lets you know when the field is disturbed and needs some clearing.

What if you do the five steps and find yourself charged up with emotional energy that just won't move on? Chances are the present-day situation has some history in old, entrenched issues. In times like this, your commitment to emotional health will require you to do some deeper detox and healing.

Emotional Healing

Learning some basics about your emotional body and feeling how e-motions work will demystify the process of feeling and healing. Tending to your emotional hygiene on a regular basis needs to be just another self-care practice. As you learned in chapter 5, blocked emotional energy means blocked physical energy. Clearing off the day-to-day is a good way to prevent illness and injury. It's also a good way to increase your emotional clarity and improve your mental focus. As you deal with surface stuff, some deeper themes will begin to emerge and ask for some deeper healing. As body-oriented therapists know, every emotional trigger has a history.

When you get your e-motions moving, does it feel like there's still more? Or does it only clear the air for a short time before everything clouds back up again? Does it seem as if your emotional story repeats itself over and over in varying scenarios? Is your idea of who you are or aspire to be restricted by old feelings and events? These are all indicators that it's time to do some emotional healing.

Like something that has been festering deep in the flesh, when your issues come to the surface, it's an opportunity to heal. When you do the work, the rewards will be great. Somatic therapists believe that the root of an emotional issue needs to be contacted and felt in order to release the stored energy. Cognitive therapists warn that if the body is saddled with an outdated message, it can distort one's self-image, influence others, and become negative self-fulfilling prophecy.[18] For instance, an old trauma might be living in your slumped posture. The resulting compression makes it difficult to feel buoyant and positive, and it can convey a message to others that you're unapproachable or in a bad mood. For bodyworkers, the connection between emotional and physical holding patterns is clear: old issues show up as current maladies.

✿ Explore: Assess Your Needs

Like your physical body, your emotional body can get bumped, scarred, hobbled, and wounded by things that happen in life. When do you know the time is right to do some emotional healing? Ask your wise body the following questions and you'll have the answer:

- Does a current situation/relationship trigger feelings/memories from the past?

- Do the five steps barely make a dent?

- Is it hard to find your emotional neutral? Is staying there impossible?

---

18 Amy Cuddy, "Your Body Language May Shape Who You Are," filmed June 2012 at TEDGlobal, 20:19, www.ted.com/amy_cuddy_your_body_language_shapes_who_you_are?share =1c7ca032el.

- Does feeling overcharged, exhausted, or numb feel normal?

- Is your voice too soft or too loud?

- Is there tension that won't let go?

- Are your joints stiff, restless, or painful?

- Do you get injured or sick repeatedly?

- Are you walking around in a turmoil, funk, or fog?

- Are your emotional responses inappropriate?

Take out your Body Wisdom journal and describe how each *yes* answer feels in your body and what emotional history might be involved. Don't be dismayed if your present day experience conjures up long-buried issues. Remember, in order to do the work you need to get to the source. Also note in your survey if there is an emotional theme that seems to be stronger and more up-front than others. If so, feel where it lives in your body and ask your muscle memory, "Why?"

Stacy. When Stacy's closest friend died, even though her heart was breaking, all she felt was anger. Rather than clearing the air, when she rocked her body to evoke the grief, her fists and jaw clenched, and she felt furious rather than sad. Wondering why anger appeared rather than sorrow, she put her hand on her jaw and asked, "What's going on?" Immediately, she recalled the time many years ago when her hamster died. Instead of comforting her sobbing body, her mom bullied her to stop, saying "If you're going to get so upset, maybe you shouldn't have any more pets." To clear the way, Stacy needed to process her feelings about being ridiculed and dismissed. Then she could find the expression to grieve both her friend and her beloved pet.

Patrick. Patrick was constantly managing the latest drama in his life. When one drama abated, another took its place. He was in survival mode and couldn't even slow down to rest. Eventually, he developed a twitch in his eye that wouldn't go away. Taking a mental wellness day and sitting in his favorite chair, it was easy to feel the discomfort and intensity of his twitching muscles. He wondered what this looked like to others and went to a mirror. The reflection clearly pointed to fear and gave him an important emotional assignment. To address the twitch, he needed to find and dislodge the fear rooted in his personal history. This, of course, took more than one day, but his eye twitch was the catalyst for emotional healing that was long overdue.

Jordan. Jordan noticed that when he said yes *(to parents, bosses, lovers, and social events) and really meant* no, *his back went into spasm. When he investigated the connection, he realized that deep inside he was angry and felt betrayed by his lack of boundaries. He was stuck in an old pattern of pleasing others and afraid to change. If he said* no, *maybe people wouldn't like him and he'd be left alone. Clearly, his back was having an emotional experience. In order to keep his back moving freely, Jordan needed to do the five steps to free up a logjam of anger and fear. Then, saying* yes *or* no *or* maybe *was simply aligned with his integrity.*

Like Stacy, Patrick, and Jordan discovered, your present circumstances could be the perfect opportunity to do some emotional healing.

Suggestions for Healing

Have you located some unresolved issues, wounds, and attitudes lodged in your body? Would you like to get started right now and clean them up and clear them out? It just so happens that, once you identify the need, you can count on the circumstances in your everyday life to coalesce around the theme. Use this synchronicity to keep your curious mind on task. For instance, when you need to free up some blocked anger, everything in your life will seem slightly aggravating. When you're backed up against an old wall of sadness, you'll gravitate to the movies, music, and stories that spark your sorrow. When you're unable to feel pride, hope, gratitude, or awe, even the song of a bird can be an invitation to feel and heal. When the timing is right, old issues can surface in the midst of a yoga class or on a ten-mile run. Use these disturbances in your emotional body as a gateway to do some e-healing.

Your five steps process works just as well on the old stuff as it does on the day-to-day. Remember, your healing is personal and private. Don't overlook the importance of setting up and cleaning up. Choose an issue that calls out to you (a current disturbance or something from your journal). Take a moment to register where and how it feels in your body. Ask, "When was the first time I felt this feeling?" and "Where else did I also encounter it?" As you focus on your issue, don't get distracted by content, storyline, and analysis. Just follow the trail and gather in all the other times you felt this way. Then, find the precise sound and gesture to match what you feel and get it all moving (don't forget the scoop, tone, and animal dancing techniques mentioned above). After your session is over, remember to take a moment and clear the entire field—all the way back.

The goal of emotional healing is to live comfortably in your own skin, in the present. When you're snagged by something that happened ten or twenty years ago (or even yesterday), your emotional experience and expression are locked in the past. It's like wearing an old suit that cramps your style and tells other people you're outdated. If it's hard to show up and stay focused in the present moment, a big overview of your emotional history can highlight where your energy is snagged. Here are some e-healing stories to inspire you:

Robert. Robert couldn't do certain tai chi moves gracefully because his body was stiff and inflexible. He noticed a similar obstruction in his personal relationships and wondered if there was an emotional source. He recalled that as a child, he tightened his muscles to feel strong whenever he felt vulnerable. Before he could let go of the armor that kept him from life and love, Robert needed to do some e-healing. Using the five steps as a template, he began to tremble first with anger and then with fear. Once he plugged into the source, it felt as if the energy moved through and out of his body like an electrical current. When he opened his mouth a sound came out that he'd never heard before. He repeated the process over the next few weeks. Each time he visited the source, the release was easier and took less time. Afterward, he was rewarded with more range in his tai chi and more resiliencies in his social life.

Lori. Every time Lori spoke with her brother, she had a heavy feeling in her chest. Afterward, she carried the disturbance into the rest of her day like a heavy, distracting burden. Rationally, Lori knew this was counterproductive and unhealthy, but emotionally she carried her family history like a wound just waiting to be prodded. She didn't feel comfortable opening the whole can of worms but was intrigued by the scoop and throw technique. When she put it into practice, Lori could feel the burden lift off her chest immediately. Curiously, using this technique consistently seemed to create a tangible distance between her emotional present and her emotional past.

Even though she hadn't "emoted," her feelings were less easily triggered. Now when her brother calls, his issues are his problem and not hers.

Mandy. When Mandy broke up with her girlfriend, she was consumed with figuring out what went wrong. As her mind obsessed over the details, her stomach tied up in knots. She was miserable and her thoughts only made her more miserable. When she came to see me to relax, I put my hand on her tummy and asked, "What sound lives here?" As she connected with her pain, Mandy emitted a soft growl. "What emotion does this sound like?" It sounded a lot like slow, rumbling anger to both of us, with a quivering underlayer of fear. Giving voice to her emotions was the key to unraveling the tension in her body and getting her e-motions flowing again. Once she got it flowing, an entire history of disappointment was ready to jump on board and move on out. Being thorough with her current e-healing meant Mandy's past emotional baggage didn't need to become part of her future.

Kelly. Kelly had tension and fluttery feelings in her stomach every time she needed to "speak truth to power." She'd spent a lifetime accommodating others and stuffing her own needs. She wanted to change this dynamic and start taking care of herself but was held captive by her own fear. However, before she could break loose and know (much less speak) her truth, she needed to bypass her defensive mind. In order to connect with her emotional body, her therapist asked if there was an animal that could represent the tone and tenor of her feelings. It so happened that recently she'd come across a dog holding a terrified bunny in his tight jaws. When she mimicked the squealing and trembling, it was the perfect reflection of her inner fear. Finding a way to express her terror and vulnerability broke the hold of silence and created a vehicle for some emotional healing. Eventually, when the fear no longer had Kelly in its clutches, it was easier to find her own power and communicate her truth.

You'll know when the e-healing happens because you can *feel* the difference. Like any load, the longer you've carried it, the heavier it is. After you've emoted, does your body feel lighter and move easier? Is your posture better and your expression freer? Has this changed your outlook and deepened your understanding? Do you feel more comfortable as an e-motional human being? Has the issue(s) that you identified in the exercise Assess Your Needs shifted or disappeared? Finding stuck or suppressed emotional energy in your body and getting it moving is a powerful way to heal your past and free up your future. It can be truly transformational.

When Self-Help Is Not Enough

When do you know that you need help? As you begin to understand the simple, physical nature of how your e-motions affect, move, and express themselves through your body, it makes a commitment to emotional hygiene and healing easier. Hopefully, this chapter has given you a fresh perspective with new ways to include and take care of your emotional body. Perhaps as part of your commitment to e-motional hygiene, you've experienced some deeper clearing and healing. As you learned more about how e-motion lives and moves in your body, you may have found complicated issues or personal history that feels intractable and hard to handle on your own. Healing a highly charged, multilayered emotional issue can take many rounds and many years to resolve. One thing is for certain, however: your emotional wounds and mega themes (abandonment, exile, betrayal, abuse, and similar) will keep showing up until you deal with them.

If any of the exercises in this chapter felt confusing, complex, or overwhelming, this could be an invitation to seek professional help. Remember, clearing emotional baggage liberates all aspects of your life and is a gift you give yourself and your future. Fortunately, more and more therapists recognize the role of the body in the equation of healing. You'll know you're with a body-oriented therapist if you are asked questions like "Where do you feel this issue in your body?" and "If your body had a voice, what would it say?" When the body is included, the underlying story and feelings are released from muscle memory and postural tension. When the body is not included, the history and issues may keep their shape long after your mind has moved on.

Evelyn. Evelyn thought her neck and shoulder tension were linked to her type-A behavior and performance anxiety. With the help of a cognitive therapist, she was able to address her issues, change her outlook, and let go of her mental tension. However, her physical tension didn't seem to budge. As she phrased it, "I feel as if I have done the psychological work but my body just hasn't gotten it yet." Her therapist urged her to look at the situation from her body's perspective. Her muscles had been doing a good job holding it all together and needed some time to relax and recalibrate. In order to embody the new agenda, Evelyn needed to get the issues out of the tissues.

A teacher, mentor, or guide can help you get out of your own way. There may be many accomplished professionals in your community who have a wide range of specialties from cognitive and talk therapy to nonverbal somatic therapies like dance therapy, authentic movement, and transformational bodywork. With so many choices, deciding where to go could feel overwhelming… so why not let your body help?

✿ *Try This: Your Body Has Some Input Too*

When seeking the right therapist/guide for your needs/situation, consider your options. Ask around and seek the good opinions of your family, friends, and colleagues. Next, take all the information and let your wise body choose: Close your eyes and visualize different paths extending in front of you, each one leading to a source of help. Imagine walking toward each possibility and notice how you feel. Perhaps approaching one path makes you feel flat and dull or anxious and foreboding. On another, perhaps the air gets thick and your body feels as if it's moving through molasses. No matter what your mind says, these paths are clearly *not* opening to you. The path that opens will feel beckoning, light-filled, and easy to approach; your body-voice will be saying yes.

A Healthy Emotional Body

Like a river, a healthy emotional body is an open channel of moving energy. As you've discovered, when the flow is slowed down, diverted, or stopped, your emotional body can feel pretty murky and toxic. Good hygiene happens when you understand the dynamic, make friends with your feelings, and keep your e-motional currents moving. This doesn't mean you're constantly emoting—far from it. When your emotional body is robust and supple, you respond to stimuli appropriately, process responsibly, and move on. Cleaning up your emotional backlog and staying in the present moment positions you for a smooth ride. And like a river, when you happen to encounter obstacles, rapids, or stormy weather, they'll just be part of your flow.

Make no mistake: your feelings are an asset. When you understand how your emotional body works and do the work to make it function optimally, it can be an intelligent and intuitive guide. Here's how three people did the work, followed their wise body, and reaped the benefits:

Ed. Ed couldn't seem to connect with his teenage daughter. Of course, some of this goes with the territory, but the situation also brought up some unprocessed grief that sat like a heavy brick on his chest. Once he put time aside to process his own feelings, he could listen to hers. Without an emotional overlay, Ed found the words, tenor, and timing to hear and support his daughter when she needed it most.

Jake. While interviewing a new person for a position at his company, Jake felt fear in the room but not in his own body. Knowing this, Jake strategically took a few moments to talk casually and create an easy environment. Instead of confronting the anxiety in the actual interview, Jake was able to get a clear idea of the candidate's interests and skill set. Trusting his emotional body helped Jake see both the fear and the person. This is the kind of emotional intelligence that makes Jake such a good boss.

Ashley. No matter how much we might plan, life can be unpredictable. A healthy emotional body can offer resilience and responsiveness in the most difficult times. When Ashley's father died, she felt as if the world had turned upside down. With so many layers of emotion and so many demanding details, her mind was in turmoil and her body was disoriented. Remembering to take some private time to be in her body and clear the feelings, she was able to find the poetry and a philosophical perspective to stand steady and stay focused. Because she'd done quite a bit of her own healing, Ashley had the clarity and confidence to help her show up for herself and her family.

Twenty-first century body wisdom tells us that if you want to claim happiness, you must also know sorrow. And if you want to be peaceful, you must embrace the turmoil of e-motion. If your emotional body is healthy, you're able to access the full spectrum of emotional experience and expression. Many people are afraid to embrace their feelings because they assume their emotions are a source of weakness and vulnerability. But when you take care of your hygiene and healing, your feeling self will be one of your greatest strengths and the foundation for emotional intelligence.

A Healthy Emotional Body Is the Key to Good Communication

Anytime your expression (postural, gestural, and facial) aligns with the message, it conveys authenticity and confidence. If you want to be trusted, you need to say yes—or no—with your body as well as your words. Communicating through the intelligence of your emotional body is good for your personal life just as it's good for business. When you pay attention to your feeling body, the timing will be spot-on when you step forward to offer an opinion, seal a deal, or make a move toward intimacy. You'll also know when to shut up and listen, finding that when you do, your smart body can tune in to what's being said (verbally and nonverbally) and deliver a message (verbally and nonverbally) that the words have been heard.

A Healthy Emotional Body Is the Key to Good Relationships

Besides communication skills, good relationships need good boundaries. Knowing your physical boundary is pretty straightforward, but knowing your emotional boundary is an accomplishment that takes some time. Once you've done the work and cleared the trauma/drama, your armor can be strong and supple rather than rigid and brittle. When you're comfortable and familiar with the boundaries of your emotional body, your sense of self can respond appropriately and help you stay safe, in control, out of conflict, and without pain. Rather than being reactive, you can be responsive and discriminatory; you know when to be close and when to keep your distance; you know when to engage and when to take a pass. Having a good relationship with your feeling self can also be lifesaving when you need to notice signals, assess danger, and respond to an emergency.

A Healthy Emotional Body Is the Key to Mastery

As many have said, growth happens and mastery is developed through the trials and tribulations of life. If you've done your work, you can be resilient and responsive when things get challenging. Instead of being thrown off your stride, you have the opportunity to stretch and perform. You can stand on the threshold of each moment instead of getting buried in the past. When you embrace the constantly moving nature of your e-motions, it's a spiritual experience akin to the Buddhist principle of impermanence. Like all things in the natural world, when a feeling crops up, you know that "this too shall pass." While it's passing, a healthy emotional body is your link to the poetry of life. Wouldn't it be boring if you had no feelings about the art you saw or music you heard? Wouldn't it be strange if you felt nothing about children or nature or creativity?

Wouldn't it be dull if the stories you heard or the stories you lived didn't resonate in your emotional body?

If you have a healthy emotional body, you can show up and experience life without getting stuck, tripped up, or held back. Now you're in the flow and ready to explore the rewards and pleasures of intimacy and intuition.

Seven
Intimacy and Intuition

There's a symbiotic relationship between intimacy and intuition. You need a strong connection to your intuition in order to be close and responsive in an intimate relationship. You need an intimate connection with yourself in order to access your intuitive resources. For both, you need to trust your body and its inner wisdom. You learn a little more about yourself and your inner resources every time you increase your body awareness, pay attention to body-talk, and follow your body-truth. Now it's time to learn about loving and being loved—knowing and being known.

The Intimacy Connection

Even before you were born, your wee body was developing a kinesthetic sense of movement, space, and relationship. Quite simply, when your mother moved, you moved and there was no separation. If your mom felt safe, you felt safe; if she was relaxed, you were relaxed. This primal, physical relationship was your first experience of intimacy. As your world expanded, your body was busy recording and storing vital information about comfort, trust, and connection. Today, those first impressions still form the baseline for your ability to experience, give, and receive intimacy.

In those early years, your infant body naturally moved toward the positive and away from the negative, just like any organism. When you were held and comforted, the world was welcoming and you opened to it. When you were neglected or stressed, you retreated. As you grew and the years went by, your body was downloading impressions and forming opinions without a word being spoken. If you felt safe and encouraged, your body moved with confidence and trust. If you felt criticized and restricted, your body learned to be cautious. Even though you may have impressive communication skills, if your circuitry is carrying negative information, it'll show up in the delicate dance of intimacy. When your body-memory is wired to the past, it might direct you to freeze, shrink, or withdraw instead of reach out, engage, and connect. The performance might look great on the outside, but *you* know if your body feels numb, distant, restricted, or distressed.

In order to clear the way for unfettered intimacy and close relationships, start with what you know. What were the circumstances or events that may have challenged or interrupted your intimacy connection? Did your conception, gestation, and birth go smoothly? Did your early life include any trauma or drama? Were you touched, hugged and held enough? Was your home a place of safety and support? Did you feel included and important? Were there times when you experienced isolation due to injury, illness, or surgery? Maybe everyone around you was busy and your needs were a low priority. Maybe your primary people had intimacy blocks of their own. If your intimacy connection is snagged on some personal history, your body wisdom can help repair the circuitry and open the channel.

🌸 Explore: Baby's New Bedtime Story

Set aside some time to go back to the very beginning and reroute the wobbly places in your birth story. Even if you don't know the particulars, just close your eyes and picture the progression. As you move from conception to gestation to birth, pay attention to your body. Does it stay relaxed, spacious, and quiet for one part of the journey and get agitated for another part? Pause at the "first light" moment and feel the presence of people awaiting your arrival. Does your body feel warm and welcome? Or, does it tighten up a bit, get fluttery, or go numb? Let your body-memory tell you what it knows. Now, take out your Body Wisdom journal and use your imagination to write a new story. Basically, you want a passage that is smooth, steady, and supportive. These are some suggestions for a good beginning:

- Conception is guided by intention, commitment, and love

- The period of gestation is safe and nurturing

- There are elements of music, poetry, touch, and words of encouragement

- A peaceful birth passage—no problems, delays, or obstructions

- The participation of key players who are focused and fully present

- A setting that supports mother and baby

- Welcoming touches and words as you enter this world

Include descriptive details that make sense to your body, such as lighting, sounds, smells, scents, and feelings. Give your story a unifying theme of trust, comfort, beauty, and support. When the continuum is seamless and positive, your bedtime story is complete. Now, find a cozy place to read it aloud to your body. Touch your heart and hear your voice come from deep inside your chest. Use your senses to feel the warmth, see the light, and receive the caress. Rock gently and relax as your body hears and absorbs the words and images. Because you've imagined it, heard it, and felt it, this story came from you and belongs to you. Hear the new story and let your body record the information. It's not that your original story disappears; it's more like you've added another memory.

Current research indicates that memory is an ongoing, creative process. What you remember has a lot to do with the story you tell about the events and effects of the past. Telling your body a new story is like planting a new set of memories.[19] When you include the elements of smell, touch, and feeling, your body records the details in its sensual experience. Because your first impressions are fundamental and set the course for the future, you want references that have positive associations. Whether it's your birth story or your life story, going back to the source helps you bring closure to the past and use your body wisdom to open up the future.

....

19   Susan Krause Whitbourne, "What Your Most Vivid Memories Say About You," in *Psychology Today,* November 20, 2012. www.psychologytoday.com/blog/fulfillment-any-age/201211 /what-your-most-vivid-memories-say-about-you.

Growing Up

Your relationship to intimacy was set at the beginning of your life and shaped by circumstances along the way. As events unfolded and things were not always perfect, they *in-formed* your understanding of how to be close, even with yourself. As an adult, your body-memory may be carrying so many qualifiers that it's hard to know what unfettered intimacy feels like. Just as your body tucked away information about riding a bicycle or holding a pencil, it has stored information about how to respond, get close, connect to, and interact with others. Of course, you want your personal history to include just the right combination of support, attachment, trust, and contact to make being intimate natural and easy. But what if the circuitry is gummed up with messages of caution or distress? Here are some body memories that can get in the way of your intimacy connection:

- If the hug/touch you needed wasn't there and your body closed off

- If you felt threatened/scared and your body tightened up

- If you were lonely/sad and your body shut down

- If there was discord/distress and your body became numb

- If there was injury/trauma and you vacated your body altogether

- If any of the above occurred and your body put up a protective shield

From your body's point of view, it makes sense to tighten, shut down, numb, disappear, or armor up in order to negotiate unpleasant, confusing, and/or painful times. From birth onward, your body has witnessed it all. Along the way, it developed management strategies and formed its own opinion about the ease, safety, and results of intimacy. You know if you have some history if you feel cautious, nervous, awkward, scared, or distracted when your body gets close to others. The bad news is if you've spent a lifetime practicing ways to protect your tender self, your body becomes good at shielding, distancing, and deflecting. But the good news is your adult perspective gives you the hindsight/insight to heal and move on. Your current-day relationships are an opportunity to heal the past and practice trusting, embracing, and showing up for intimacy. The best place to start is your relationship with yourself.

Self-Love

On some level, every single exercise in this book has been about self-love. As you've discovered, even if you want to show up for love, it's hard to do if your body is holding back. To receive a comforting hug, a tender touch, or encouraging words, it's helpful if your body is open and receptive. To initiate intimacy with others, it's helpful if your body feels confident and self-assured. In order to love others, you need to love yourself. Here's what self-love looks like:

- You feel at one with your body

- You trust your body and include it in decision-making

- It's easy to find three or four things you like about your body

- You show up appropriately and authentically for tough times

- You feel at home in your body and are comfortable being alone

- You have a sense of belonging and feel connected

- You move in your world with confidence

If any of these basics aren't easy for you, the place to start on your quest for intimacy is with your own body. What does this look like in everyday terms? It means you tune in and check in frequently. It means you care for your body's needs as lovingly as you would a dear friend or pet. You don't dismiss, override, suppress, or deride your body. Rather, you encourage, acknowledge, include, and honor it. When you love yourself, it feels natural to be held, heard, touched, and respected by others.

❀ Try This: Give Yourself a Little Love

Bring your hands to a part of your body that gets little attention, such as your elbows, knees, or the back of your head. Settle in, get comfortable, and let your touch soften, mold, and make full contact with the contour, shape, and warmth of your body. Stay in contact for a few minutes as you get to know this part.

- *Touch* your body as if it were innocent and precious, like a baby

- *Communicate* a message of love and high regard

- *Dissolve* the interface between your hand/body and let two parts become one

- *Connect* with the essence of flesh, bone, and pulse of life that resides here

How did it feel to get intimate and give your body a little love? At first, did the exercise feel strange? Did you want to hurry up and get it over with? Did you encounter any hesitation, awkwardness, self-judgment, or emotion? Did your body seem distant, disconnected, or unfamiliar? Any time you touch or care for your physical body (feeding, dressing, bathing, massaging, and so on), you can give/receive a little love just by slowing down and being present. Most people find that it takes some time and practice to undo the negative spin about touching consciously and lovingly, but it's a worthy cause.

❀ *Try This: Ask for a Hug*

Receiving a hug increases your capacity for closeness and augments your feel-good physiology. Why not put it to the test and see what happens? For the next week, engage a hugging partner. It could be a good friend, a pet, or even a pillow. Once a day, line up with as much body contact as possible (head to the right, left ear to left ear, heart to heart). Just be there and stay there for a count of seven seconds. No squeezing, swaying, patting, or chatting. After each hugging session, take a moment to evaluate the experience. How did your body respond? Did you feel some tension leave? Were you self-conscious, awkward, embarrassed, apologetic, or uneasy? Was it hard to just be present without doing anything? Did any feelings or memories come up? Did you become a better hugger as you got more practice? Did you learn something about nonsexual intimacy? What did your hugging partner experience?

Although this exercise was more about receiving than giving, rest assured your hugging partner got some goodies as well. Several studies suggest that one little hug increases a powerful hormone/neurotransmitter, oxytocin, called the "love drug" that is credited for:

- Increasing trust

- Promoting feelings of optimism

- Improving self-esteem

- Reducing social anxiety and inhibition[20]

As a result of your hugging sessions, did you notice any of these qualities carry through to other parts of your life? It's easy to see how a daily dose of the "love drug" could augment your intimacy connection.

> *Pattie. Pattie had never felt totally at ease around other people, so it came as no surprise that the seven-second-hug exercise was challenging. Even though her mind felt safe, her body had to override the urge to break away. However, after a couple of days' practice, she noticed something shift. Halfway through the hug, her body tension softened and being close felt more natural. The experience even started to feel somewhat pleasurable. Over the week, Pattie's hugging ability improved and her body could move close and sustain intimacy from beginning to end. Consequently, she felt more socially assured for the rest of the day. As a result of a simple hugging experiment, she'd found a way to stay in her body and connect with others with grace and confidence.*

Self-love is about showing up, without hesitation, to receive. Notice what happens when someone gives you help, attention, pleasure, love, or gifts. Does your body get tight, fidgety, uncomfortable, or numb? Maybe this is why they say it's easier to give than receive. To establish a good intimacy connection, you may need to practice receiving.

✿ *Explore: Get a Massage*
Schedule a therapeutic massage to practice the art of receiving. In this setting, all you need to do is show up, be yourself, and notice what happens. Some things you might observe could be:

....
20   "The Power of Love—Hugs and Cuddles Have Long-term Effects," in *NIH News in Health*, February 2007, newsinhealth.nih.gov/2007/february/docs/01features_01.htm.

- How easy or difficult it is to focus on your body when it's receiving

- How challenging it is for your arms, legs, head to let go

- Some parts feel familiar, comfortable, estranged, or awkward

- Any emotional content or unconscious resistance

- Physiological signs of anxiety or dis-ease; pleasure or healing

- How your mind keeps interrupting and diverting your attention

- Self-criticism or old messages that pop up

When a subtext appears during a massage, let it go and come back to your muscles, organs, and bones. Be in your body, in the room, and in the moment. Afterward, you can write it all down in your journal. How long were you able to stay focused before your mind took you away? What issues or feelings or considerations came up? What insights or information did your body have for you? If this experience had something to teach you about your body, make a few more appointments. Like the seven-second hug, you'll find being on the receiving end of a massage easier and easier. Someday, it'll just feel natural to receive care and attention.

Loving Others
Being at home in your own body makes it easier to feel at home with others. Just showing up 100 percent in your body puts you in contact with the moment, person, and place. Because intimacy is a simple process of giving and receiving, it can happen in many different contexts: with a friend, in nature, enjoying art, playing with a pet, or being at an event. A degree of intimacy can happen while standing next to someone at a political rally or making eye contact in the supermarket. It's possible to feel an intimate connection any time, at any place: quiet your mind, stay in your body, and be in the moment.

Throughout this book, you've learned how to respect and live in your wise body. Understanding how your body communicates helps you be true to yourself and authentic with others. Knowing how to spot and handle emotional content gives you good boundaries and social acumen. You've given it the test and your body has proven to be a good resource for good relationships. All of this comes in handy when it comes to exploring intimacy. Loving others is much easier if you know how to open your heart, be sensible, and share space.

Open Your Heart

Your emotions affect your heart. Anger and irritation make your blood pressure rise and long-term aggravation can result in a permanent state of hypertension. When you feel loss, pain, or sorrow, the heart space becomes tight, achy, or heavy. When you feel resentment, jealousy, or judgment, it gets blocked and constricted. When you feel safe, you expand; when you don't feel safe, you contract. You can feel it in your chest. See what happens in your body when you even think about something emotionally painful or disturbing. Notice how your chest muscles tighten when you encounter a threat or surprise. These are reliable responses if emotion is fresh and a threat is nearby, but if your instinct to protect becomes a permanent feature, it makes it hard to give and receive love.

Many people believe that the heart is the center of emotional empathy and acceptance of others. When your heart is open, you're open to unconditional love. When you feel self-worth and a high regard for others, the heart space becomes filled with lightness, hope, and joy. This is as much about the body as it is about the mind.

❀ Try This: Get Big-Hearted

Take a moment to close your eyes and touch the center of your sternum with your fingers. Feel the back of your body touch the chair at the same latitude. Now focus on the area between front and back. This is your heart space. As you breathe into your heart space (filling and emptying, front and back), let the movement loosen up any stillness/holding/tension. As you exhale, release all jealousy, worry, dissatisfaction, judgment, and so on. As you inhale, fill with love and acceptance. Can you feel your heart space soften and expand? On your next exhale, send some caring compassion to the significant people in your life. Does getting big-hearted give you a benevolent connection to something greater than your small self?

If your heart space is relaxed, giving and receiving is easy. When you show up with an open heart, other people are invited to show up and open up as well. Your open heart is the doorway to an intimacy that goes well beyond a one-on-one relationship. As spiritual teachers have said in different ways: open your heart to the beauty and perfection of the universe and you can feel at one with all there is.

Be Sensible

Like many people, your dominant mode may be what you think rather than what you feel, hear, smell, etc. Whenever I ask someone where they live in their body, the answer is always, "in my head." However, they aren't talking about their body-head (chin-cheeks-forehead)—they really mean their thinking head. If your awareness has been corralled by cognitive thinking 24/7, it takes some practice to shift gears and be *sensible* for intimacy. The case isn't hard to make: if you're off thinking or fantasizing or figuring things out, you won't be available to feel, give, *or* receive. To show up for intimacy, your awareness needs to be in the room, in your body, and nowhere else.

❀ *Try This: Everyday Intimacy*

When you're tuned in to your senses, even mundane activities can feel intimate, so just show up and pay attention. Let the routine things you do every day help you learn about giving and receiving. Nothing changes except your focus when you:

- Wash your face and feel the smoothness of your skin

- Smell a rose and enjoy the pleasure of its scent

- Hear the wind in the chimes or birdsong and let the sound fill the moment

- Walk and feel the delight of your hips swaying/legs moving/ arms swinging

- Taste a mouthful of food and linger to savor the flavor

- Float on your back and feel the caress of the water

Why do you think humans are drawn to velvet and silk, perfumed scents and a warm bath, sweet melodies and chocolate? Such sensual pleasures help you feel *in touch*. When you bring your sensible body along, even the most casual situation can feel intimate and meaningful. Not only do you sense the essence of experience, but you pick up the nuances of nonverbal communication that are vital for successful relationships. When you're interacting with others, here's what your sensible body might be telling you:

- Feeling warm and relaxed: safety, comfort, go ahead

- Muscles that feel hesitant/tight/jumpy: caution, slow down

- A sense of erogenous activity: there's sexual energy (yours/theirs)

- Hearing or eyesight seems dull/flat/blocked: change course/stop

- Feeling spaced out or unfocused: distraction/no connection

In a nutshell, if your sensible body feels fluid and expansive, you can proceed with confidence. If it shuts down and contracts, you'd be wise to slow down, create some distance, or hold off for now. If it tenses up, checks out, feels uneasy, or has any other reaction, this is important feedback. Use these signals to determine the pace and tenor of your relationships. If you override your senses every once in a while and push ahead anyway, don't overlook the consequences. It's all part of learning.

Tune In to Personal Space

Basically, your innate sense of space sets your boundaries—where you end and the world around you begins. Throughout this book you've been encouraged to pay attention to your spacious body—how it feels, how it moves, and how it connects. Being space savvy means you're aware of the biofield beyond your body. This seemingly empty space actually contains electromagnetic vibrations that are influenced by where you are and how you feel. This personal exterior space helps you keep your integrity as you relate to others.

The size of your biofield is influenced by moods and circumstances. When you feel good, it expands; when you feel exuberant, it really expands. Accordingly, it shrinks when you feel depressed, scared, cautious, or unwelcomed. It contracts when you want to deflect unwanted attention, and expands when you want to include others in your bubble of intimacy. You can feel this practical resiliency if you compare the amount of personal space you occupy in different situations, such as riding in a crowded subway, sitting with a loved one, standing near a volatile person, or lying in a field of daisies.

🌸 *Try This: How Much Personal Space Do You Need?*

Your personal space doesn't end at your skin. It generally extends four to eight inches beyond your body in what is called your *biofield* or *energy field*. Close your eyes and check this out. Feel how your personal space radiates beyond your body. Does your bio-field feel big or small? Your personal space varies depending on mood and circumstance. Sometimes it can get really big and fill a room; other times it can shrink right up close to your body. Check out how big you feel when you're happy, hopeful, satisfied, and comfortable. Contrast this with how small you feel when you're depressed, scared, tired, or focused on a problem. Does your energy field expand to include others when you feel safe? Does it put up a shield when you don't? Even though you can't see it, your energy field is powerful. And even though others can't see your energy field, it has an influence. Have you noticed how others keep their distance when you're disturbed or distracted? Conversely, do you notice how you attract attention when you feel expansive and gregarious?

If you're feeling relaxed, open, and welcoming, it's easy to share space with others. Unfortunately, regardless of intention or desire, if your personal space is hardwired for defense, it won't be easy to let others in. Does being close and staying close always feel awkward, distracting, uncomfortable, or threatening? This can be a result of your personal history or the circumstances of habit. When you're locked into a fast-paced, high-tech, chaotic, urban lifestyle, intimacy creates a challenge. In a physical sense, you need to know how to soften defenses in order to be close and inclusive. To explore the intimacy of sharing space, you'll want to start with something simple and uncomplicated.

🌸 *Explore: Feel the Intimacy of Place*

The best way to become acquainted with your energy field is sitting alone, away from the madding crowd. This could be in the quiet sanctuary of your bedroom or in a special place out in nature (in the woods, on an isolated stretch of beach, halfway up a mountain trail, or near a tree in your backyard). Close your eyes and get comfortable. Quiet your mind and body. Give yourself enough time to come thoroughly into the present moment. Then observe your intimate connection to the air above and around your head, the ground under your feet. This is your personal space. Now, extend your sense of space to include the surrounding flora, fauna, sky and earth. Feel the touch of air, smell the earth and plants, hear the birds and bees. Let your space-savvy sensual body become intimate with your surroundings. What does this feel like? In this moment, your presence is a part of the scene. Can you sustain this intimacy of place for a bit?

Even if you didn't feel any connection at all beyond your feet touching the earth, give yourself credit for being intimate with the spot right under your feet. Learning how to share space can teach you a lot about yourself. Take out your Body Wisdom journal and record your experience, challenges, discoveries, and insights. Draw a picture of your expanded energy field comingling with all the life around.

Once you're familiar with the basics of self-love and loving others, your intimacy connection is plugged in and ready to go. You're ready for the adventure. Being body wise adds a whole new dimension to the most complicated, challenging, and rewarding aspect of human experience—intimacy.

Intimacy Practicum

Now it's time to do some field work so you can become a master of the intimate moment. An intimate moment can happen in a split second in eye contact at a tollbooth or be extended for hours making love to your partner. When you understand that intimacy covers a wide range of experience and a broad scope of possibilities, you'll find lots of opportunities to practice your skills. Just listen to your wise body.

How are you communicating?

Intimacy is about communication. You pick up and respond to nonverbal signals all the time. When you pay attention to the subtleties of what's going on, you can gauge the degree of appropriate intimacy for the situation. If your tone and gestures match the situation, communication becomes both more effective and more intimate. For instance, if you pick up sorrow, you soften a bit. If you pick up excitement, you increase the tempo. If you sense hesitation, you slow down. Additionally, when you pay attention to nonverbal cues, you know how your communication is going. For example, if you observe open and relaxed gestures, you may assume that all's going well. If eyes glaze over, there's no interest. If arms are crossed and jaw set, there's resistance. You know if your listener is critical because you feel your own guard go up. You know if you're not connecting because no matter how many people are in the room, you feel alone. And all of this information gets delivered without a word being spoken. Receptivity, appreciation, and agreement are part of nonverbal communication.

❀ Try This: Body-Talk

Body-talk (eye contact, gesture, expression, and emotional tenor) tells you what's really going on. As you interact with people over the next few days, tune in to the subliminal message. Listen with your eyes as well as your ears to *see* what's being said. Do the words match the body talk? Look at the person's mouth, eyes, and hands; check out the movement of their head and demeanor of posture. Do you see receptivity and agreement or disinterest and opposition? What do the tone and tempo tell you? Perhaps an upbeat delivery is broadcasting optimism or joy. Slumped shoulders and a downcast expression may indicate a pensive, distracted mood. Take a chance and trust your interpretation. Next, match your own volume/gestures/tone/tempo and feel the effect. When you include nonverbal communication, do you connect more intimately with the person and the moment?

❀ Try This: Listening Is Part of the Conversation

This fun experiment will show you how important physical presence is for intellectual intimacy. Get together with a friend and set it up alternately so that one person talks about something of interest while the other person listens. At a random moment, the listener will tighten around the solar plexus (gut) and cross his/her arms. Check out how this slight shift influences the quality of communication. Did the speaker feel less fluid, more inhibited, less intimate? Did the listener feel distracted or disengaged? Now switch positions and see how the other side feels. In order to show up for the conversation, your body has to be there. In order for intimacy to happen, you both have to be there.

Deanna. Deanna is a good boss. Although she has many employees, she strives to see and relate to each one individually. She does this not by knowing names or recalling particulars, but through her physical presence. By including body-talk in the dialogue, she's able to make an intimate connection and communicate with clarity. For instance, if an employee is enthusiastic and upbeat, Deanna matches the tempo. If he/she is leaning forward/backward, Deanna does the same. If the tone is soft, she responds softly. When the boss puts her intimacy skills to work, not only does she receive more information about her employees, but they in turn feel heard and seen. As an effective employer, she's seen how to engender trust and cooperation through nonverbal communication.

Tips for Good Communication

Being able to read and respond to body-talk is an important part of your emotional intelligence. Here are some ways to increase your communication skills and improve your intimacy connection.

- Speak from the heart. Literally, let your voice come from mid-chest. This gives your tone a quality of engagement and authenticity.

- When you want to be understood, connect with your base (feet, pelvis). This will ground your words' conviction and confidence.

- When you want to communicate receptivity, keep your hands open and relaxed. This tells the speaker that you're present and attentive.

- Make eye contact for direct conversations; stand side by side for casual, less intense interactions

- If you want to speak to the emotional/intuitive aspect of someone, look into the left eye (wired to the right brain); if you want to speak to the analytical/rational aspect of someone, look into the right eye.

- When you want to gauge the feeling/tone, remember to observe the facial and postural expressions.

How's Your Focus?

Intimacy requires your undivided attention. Some degree of intimate connection occurs in any aware moment. But in order to show up and *be* in the moment, you need mental focus. Let's be honest, you can't be entirely present if your mind is surfing several channels at once. Unfortunately, like most people, your mind might be so habitually distracted that you never show up 100 percent of the time. When you read a story to a six-year-old, hug your sweetie, or go to a concert with a friend, is your mind busy elsewhere? As you discovered in chapter 1, you can use your body-centered awareness (breathing, touching, seeing, hearing, smelling) to quiet your busy mind and focus on the present moment.

Over the next few days, observe your thought process in even the most casual, mundane conversations. Notice how your focus wanders while dining with a colleague, chatting with a neighbor, or catching up with loved ones. Does your mind chatter endlessly, multitask, or jump ahead to your next comment? Once you check out the quality of your focus, bring your attention to your body. Feel how the measured tempo of your breath moves your ribs; sense the weight of your pelvis on the chair and the touch of your feet on the ground. Instead of filling the interior space with language and random thoughts, let your head just be the top part of your body. Now, see how long you keep your focus on the present moment and all it has to offer. Remember, the quality of an intimate moment is determined by who shows up.

❋ Try This: An Intimate Dinner Alone

The next time you sit down to eat, let go of everything and simply *be here now*. Notice where and how you're sitting. Feel your feet on the ground. Make adjustments so you're supported, balanced, and comfortable. As you partake of the meal, observe the smell, taste, and presentation of the food. Don't name or evaluate or compare—just let it register in your senses. Keep your focus on the physical experience of the meal and the moment. Notice—and resist—the urge to look at your phone, read a newspaper, watch TV, make lists, ponder a problem, or just space out. Notice what happens when your mind wanders away from the moment. Your body may still be at the table, but *you* aren't. When you sharpen your focus and experience the flavor and texture, even partaking of a simple orange can be an intimate experience.

❋ Try This: Sharing Silence

You might be surprised to hear that some cultures value silence as a way to connect. In our culture, being silent can feel disturbing, intimidating, scary, awkward, or simply wrong. Get a friend to join you and check out what happens when you walk or sit next to each other for a few minutes of focused silence. Instead of filling the space with talk, just breathe and be quietly present. Then check in with your companion and share your experiences. Did the silence feel intolerable or awkward? Did your mind rush in to fill the space with internal chatter, judgments, or feelings? Did some old emotions and self-talk show up that you might want to process later? Without conversation, did your mind wander out of the shared space? Did your body feel jittery, self-conscious, or shy? Like anything new and different, the more you practice, the more comfortable you'll feel sharing silence. Of course, this can be easier to practice if you're also sharing an activity like planting a garden, riding the chairlift, or hiking a mountain trail.

You can sharpen your ability to focus anywhere (e.g., in the classroom, boardroom, living room, or bedroom). How you show up sets the stage. When you clear your mind and center your awareness in present time, your intimacy connection is plugged in and ready to go. When your mind is cluttered or your attention is somewhere else, the connection is full of static. Remember that intimacy doesn't have to be about physical touch or romance. Empty your multitasking, wandering, distracted mind and let your focused presence create a context for intimacy.

In order to experience any degree of intimacy, you need to show up mentally as well as physically. Here are some ways to augment your focusing ability and improve your intimacy connection:

- Practice meditation. Being able to keep your awareness in the present moment takes practice.

- When you listen, just listen. Don't fill your head space with internal conversation or ponder your next comment while someone else is speaking. If you want to be in a relationship you need to pay attention.

- Stay in your body. Make sure your body-talk matches the words and the words match your intention.

- Slow down. You don't need to figure out what happens next in order to get there. Measuring your cadence by the tempo of your breath will help you stay in the flow.

- Wherever you are, be there 100 percent.

Are You a Sensitive Person?

Intimacy is about sensitivity. Being a sensitive person means you're aware of your feelings and the feelings of others. Paying attention to the emotional body helps you decode the subtle undertones and adapt accordingly. The delicate duet of intimacy is much easier when you get the whole picture.

A sensitive person is touched, moved, or impressed by people, circumstances, and events without being thrown off. A sensitive person detects the subtle cues and responds appropriately, and their detection happens without saying a single word. For example, if a situation calls for compassion and caring, you might want to extend a gentle touch, a knowing glance, or a nod of the head. Many times, this is more effective than a direct reference. At the same time, of course, other people are receiving information directly from your emotional body. Anytime there's a subtext (yours or theirs), you can increase trust and intimacy when you include emotion-based words (e.g., *awkward, hard, painful, scary, exciting,* and so on) to own how you're feeling. Being sensitive to others' emotional tenor can personalize a brief encounter in the supermarket, an intense negotiation in the boardroom, or a tricky discussion with a loved one.

Suzanne. Suzanne and her eighteen-year-old son kept going around and around the same issue. She felt shut out; he felt smothered. Mother and son couldn't find the words to get through, and neither felt heard. Both were trying to defend positions intellectually without owning the underlying feelings. Finally, Suzanne shifted her perspective from her intellect to her emotional body and found a way through the impasse. She said to her son, "When you exclude me from your life, I feel sadness in the pit of my stomach. Let's figure out a way where I can feel included without crowding you." Referencing the body made Mom's statement both authentic and nonconfrontational. It also set the tone for her son's response, "When you 'helicopter' around me, it makes me panic. Even if you don't say a thing, your opinions are loud and clear. I need some distance in order to hear my own voice and find my own power." Being sensitive created the context for this honest, intimate sharing. It also opened the door for future trust and understanding.

❀ *Try This: Staying Calm*

When a lover, friend, relative, or colleague erupts emotionally, do you feel their panic, confusion, tension, and fear in your body? Even if it has nothing to do with you, emotional fallout can be unsettling and disorienting. Although you may want to run away or find a distraction, staying consciously present and nonreactive is part of your intimacy practicum. Try some of the following strategies for being centered, confident, and compassionate when their emotions are triggered and yours aren't:

- If someone is sad, slow down and soften your approach

- If someone is animated with excitement, ramp up a bit

- If someone is forceful or angry, tighten your boundaries and step back

- If someone delivers a verbal tirade, just breathe through it and let it go

- If someone is suffering/grieving, a gentle touch conveys compassion

This is the time to remember the body basics. Eye contact is about being seen; listening is about being heard; and sharing breath is about being connected. Furthermore, your sense of space helps you determine where you end and they begin. With good boundaries, a sensitive person knows how to be present without taking on someone else's stuff. Listen to your sensitive body. It will help you identify and respond appropriately to the affect (feelings) in any tricky situation. You really don't need to do or say anything. Just showing up *without* getting reactive creates a bond of intimacy.

> *Naomi. Naomi's mom lost her beloved dog to cancer and needed a shoulder to cry on. When Naomi tried to be proactive and comforting, she was surprised to discover that doing nothing was doing something. Any attempt to distract, make suggestions, or give reassurance simply felt hollow and mismatched for this raw time. It was the shoulder her mom needed, not a solution. As she embraced and listened to her sobs, Naomi's nonreactive, nonjudgmental sensitivity helped her stay relaxed and emotionally present. When it was over, there were no words necessary except* thank you. *Mother and daughter had shared a very intimate time and it was all about being present. Sometimes the most sensitive thing you can do is bear witness.*

If there's emotion in the air, your body knows it. When you get the whole picture, you can decode emotional information and adjust your behavior accordingly. Here are some ways your sensitive body registers an emotional undertone:

- A quiver of nervous energy in your gut saying that someone nearby is anxious

- Your chest getting heavy when you hear a sad story or sense someone in grief

- Words sound hollow when the truth isn't being told

- You smell a strong, acrid odor if someone is scared

- Your body tenses up when you hear a mixed message or insincere praise

- Your erogenous zones perk up if someone is sending a sexual vibe

- Your muscles armor up around people who are judgmental or critical

- You feel relaxed around people who are loving and compassionate

When you're sensitive you get the subtext—what's going on and what's going on behind the scenes. Your wise body helps you understand the subtle messages that tell you when to move forward and when to create a bit more space, when to initiate and when to take a pass, and how to be responsive to the present situation. Being sensitive can make or break your intimacy connection. If you doubt the message or the interpretation, take a chance and ask for clarification. It's all part of your intimacy practicum.

Sharing Space

Intimacy is about shifting the epicenter from "me" to "we." Whatever the circumstance, anytime you show up, pay attention, and connect, you're sharing space. This can happen in bed with a lover, at a restaurant with a friend, in the hammock with a sleepy cat, on a marathon with fellow athletes, or at a rally with a crowd. A certain energetic intimacy occurs with close proximity whether you know it or not. People who see energy fields report that auras merge into one hue when people share space and experience. Have you ever experienced a sense of *oneness* at a sporting event, a megachurch service, or a political convention? Have you ever felt an intimate bond result from a shared road trip or traumatic event?

Sharing space isn't about losing your sense of self. It's about occupying the center and the field at the same time. You don't disappear; you just get bigger. Sharing space means you stay present, keep your focus, tune in your senses, and expand your range of intimacy. But before you expand your personal space to include others, it's important to know where you end and others begin.

❋ Try This: Walking Together

Get a friend and go for a walk where there is plenty of lateral space such as a park, playing field, or gym. Begin walking next to each other, letting the swing of your arms and legs synchronize into an easy rhythm. Walk along for a bit until you feel *together*. Then gradually increase the distance between you and your friend. Notice when it begins to feel as if you are walking alone and stop. Did you and your friend stop at about the same time? How much space did it take to feel alone? Now move gradually closer until you're in each other's physical presence again. Now get a little too close and notice how this feels. Find the perfect distance where you feel comfortable *and* together. When you show up and tune in, your sense of space is part of your intimacy connection.

❋ Try This: Public Intimacy

The next time you're attending a performance or presentation, practice sharing space. See if you can feel the group energy align after a few minutes. This shared experience becomes a kind of collective intimacy. Can you feel what the psychics see? A good performance or speaker not only connects with the audience, they connect the audience with each other. You feel the influence of this group dynamic in your body when something triggers agreement or satisfaction and everyone responds in sync. You also feel the group sync when it responds to something unpleasant or disrespectful. Can you feel the energy ricochet through your body and around the room? Do you notice the unifying force of collective disappointment when you show up and (figuratively) the speaker/performer doesn't?

Consciously sharing space not only feels good, it adds a poetic quality to being alive. If you feel safe and comfortable, you can expand your experience and explore your intimacy connection anywhere. Try it out in the supermarket or under the starry skies. Try it out at home and let your personal energy field include the whole room and everything in it. Sharing space in such a grand way brings you into relationship with all life, all that is. This can be invaluable when you're with someone who is dying, distressed, or recovering from a traumatic event. In such delicate times, your spatial presence gives you a way to show up without being overwhelmed or overwhelming. Intimacy is not always about being expressive. Sometimes, intimacy is just about *being*. Sharing space is sharing grace.

Try This: Intimate Breathing

Intimacy of spirit happens anytime you're in close proximity to another person and, without words or action, share expanded space. Breathing together is a delightful way for couples to experience intimacy and deepen their connection. Here's how:

Create a time and place to be quiet and close. Find that cozy spot where you can lie down next to each other without touching. Spend a few minutes relaxing and letting your own breath become easy and full. At the beginning, notice how your separate bodies occupy their own time and space. Then, without effort, let your sense of space expand to include the other person. Let the tension and distance between your bodies melt. Then gradually synchronize your breathing so you share the same inhale/exhale rhythm. Feel how the two breaths become one. Keep focusing on shared space/breath and let this intimacy bubble get really big. Is it hard to tell where one body ends and the other one begins? Pretty intimate, isn't it?

Try This: Sensual Intimacy

In the vernacular, being intimate often has sexual connotations. But true physical intimacy is more than attraction and sexual excitement. When sex is intimate, it's about your wise body knowing how to show up, stay aware, respond to cues, be authentic, and sustain sensual focus. It's about being expansively comfortable and expressively loving in the presence of another. It sounds complicated but it's simply about being conscious in your sensual body. Showing up and sharing space improves your intimacy and your pleasure. The next time you're feeling sexual, bring your sensual body along and practice all your intimacy skills. Keep your mind in the moment and follow the lead of your body. Expand your spatial awareness and invite the intimate moment to carry you beyond the mundane to connect with the cosmos. You'll know the moment you get there.

Your perspective has a lot to do with your comfort and ability to be close with others. Sharing space has both a physical *and* a spiritual dimension. Here are some ways to improve your intimacy connection:

- Empower your energy field. Tune in and trust the feedback. Even when you expand space to include others, your comfort level helps you discriminate positives/negatives and adjust your boundaries accordingly. (Learn more about this in chapter 8.)

- Let intimacy include your compassionate heart. This gives you a loving context for sharing intimate space even with strangers.

- Be scientific. Let your field get so big that you *are* more space than matter and part of the whole—microcosm to macrocosm.

- Get philosophical. Let quantum physics introduce you to metaphysics. Your physical experience can connect you to the oneness of all life. When two people feel as one, it can be your link to big space.

- Get spiritual. The feeling of oneness renders any moment intimate. This can be a powerful antidote for feeling estranged, alone, disconnected, or existential. Get quiet enough and big enough to let the *om* vibration be your intimacy connection.

Everything you do to improve your intimacy connection lays the foundation for reliable, body-centered intuition. Knowing how to share space is the key to an intimate relationship with your inner knowing. People who play in a jazz ensemble or dance the samba know about the link between intimacy and intuition. A competitive athlete friend describes how this works: "When I'm playing volleyball, it often feels as if I'm a part of the collective body of players. It feels like my *body* knows what will happen next." Anytime you feel connected to a place, person, event, or experience, the wiring is in place for intuition. You can sense what's happening and what's going to happen next. This is not something your mind knows, it's something your body knows.

The Intuition Connection

Intuition is the ability to know something without conscious reasoning. Your intuition serves a very important function in your life as both guardian and guide. As guardian, it looks out for your health and survival. As guide, it points the way to fulfillment and success. Even though your intuition is not part of your rational mind, it's best when they work together. Once your smart mind learns to listen to your smart body, you can trust your inner knowing to help you make decisions, connect, explore, create, experiment, take risks, and find meaning in it all. Very often, it is intuition that leads you beyond the known answers to hidden solutions. Perhaps this is why Einstein valued it so much.[21]

Intuition spans a spectrum from instinct to clairvoyance. Instinct is basic. Cells in a petri dish will move away from a harmful stimulus and toward a beneficial one. As you go through life, you encounter various pleasure/pain and success/failure experiences that condition your body's automatic responses. Just think of the old adage "once bitten, twice shy." This instinctual knowing is geared toward safety, survival, and success in the physical world. But your body has another kind of knowing that is equally innate. It is commonly referred to as *extrasensory perception* (ESP) and lies outside the field of everyday perception like seeing with eyes, hearing with ears, or feeling with skin. For instance, without thinking about it, you have a dream that something's going to happen; you get goose bumps at a significant point in a story; you think of someone just before they call; or a phrase pops into your mind that answers a question.

What's your personal experience with inner knowing? Maybe without naming it, a large part of your body wisdom *is* intuition. Haven't many of the exercises in this book asked you to tune in, listen to, and trust your body? Each time you encountered a random memory, a sudden a-ha! moment, or a significant sensation that precipitated deeper understanding, you were making an intuitive connection. Each time you trusted

....

21   Michele and Robert Root-Bernstein, "Einstein on Creative Thinking," in *Psychology Today,* March 31, 2010. www.psychologytoday.com/blog/imagine/201003/einstein-creative-thinking -music-and-the-intuitive-art-scientific-imagination.

and followed your body wisdom, you were reinforcing this conduit for inner knowing. But the proposition that you receive extrasensory information and move to action without conscious reasoning can baffle the logical mind. Here are some recent discoveries that describe some aspects of your inner knowing:

- Scientists have measured signals from the gut and heart that affect biological systems without ever looping through the brain[22]

- Experiments with the endocrine system demonstrate how behavior is influenced by smells you don't "smell" with your nose[23]

- Brain imaging shows in color what happens at the very moment of insight or inspiration[24]

- Emotions directly affect the heart[25]

- There is still that petri dish where, without prior stimulation of any kind, cells avoid pain and approach pleasure[26]

ESP: Your Inner Senses

Information from your eyes, ears, tongue, and belly registers in your brain, telling you what's going on and what to do. The stimulus-response from these regular senses is pretty obvious. But what if you could see, hear, feel, and know things without using your eyes, ears, fingers, and cognitive mind? In the jargon of ESP, this would be clairvoyance (seeing), clairaudience (hearing), and precognition (knowing). Although often deemed

....

22 Root-Bernstein, "Einstein on Creative Thinking."

23 Catherine De Lang, "The Unsung Sense: How Smell Rules Your Life," in *New Science,* September 2011. www.newscientist.com/article/mg21128301-800-the-unsung-sense-how -smell-rules-your-life.

24 Jonah Lehrer, "The Eureka Hunt," in *New Yorker,* July 28, 2008. www.newyorker.com /magazine/2008/07/28/the-eureka-hunt.htms.

25 Ibid.

26 Gloria Taraniya Ambrosia, "The Experience of Feeling," in Barre Center for Buddhist Studies, Spring newsletter 2000. www.bcbsdharma.org/article/the-experience-of-feeling-insight-into -the-aggregates/.

a pseudoscience, for the past twenty years serious researchers have used advances in medical imaging and technology to track and record ESP. Today scientists are validating what psychics and paranormal psychologists have been saying for years, that we have inner senses that are wired and ready to go. Here are a few ways you make an intuitive connection every day:

- Feeling love, hate, sexual availability, admiration, danger, and the pain of others, even with your eyes and ears closed

- Sensing if someone is sneaky, duplicitous, manipulative, or distracted

- Picking up whether someone is authentic, supportive, powerful, or honest

- Assessing a stranger's emotional state and physical health just by being in the same room

- Getting goose bumps when something is important or waves of fatigue when something is pointless

❀ *Explore: Your ESP File*

Write down any experiences you can remember that had an *extrasensory* component in your Body Wisdom journal. Over the next few days, invite your inner senses to add to this list. Make a note of the ways you receive signals and information from your intuition connection. Experiment with ESP in crowded spaces, such as public transportation, a park, an auditorium, or a school meeting. Close your eyes briefly and expand your field to include the people around you. Can you pick up discord or excitement, sorrow or fear? Do you feel a spike of emotional energy moving through your body for no reason? Take a moment to speculate where this is coming from and why. Stay playful and imaginative—you're not making a case for anything. Intuitively, emotional vibes are the easiest to pick up. Other ways your body's ESP might show up is when you:

- Think of someone just before they call

- Listen to your gut/heart when making decisions

- Use your inner knowing to assess intention and authenticity

- Respond to a sinking, hollow, or spiky feeling and take action

- Know when to shut up/speak up because your throat closes off/opens

- Experience the synchronicity of coincidence

Write down your observations in your journal as simple happenstance without any explanation, opinion, or judgment. Remember, it's not about the accuracy of your extrasensory perceptions; it's about exploring the circuitry.

Kim. Several years ago, at a resort in the Colorado Rockies, Kim trusted an intuitive impulse and avoided a tragedy. He had taken his dog out for a walk on a peaceful star-filled night. All of a sudden, the air around him seemed to stand still, he got goose bumps on his arms, and just knew something bad was going to happen. He didn't stop to doubt or take time to evaluate. He just acted on his gut feelings and pulled his dog to the side of the road. Minutes later, a car appeared out of nowhere and roared past, barely missing Kim and his dog. Once his heart stopped pounding, Kim realized that his intuition (precognition) had saved both himself and his dog from certain injury, if not death.

Everyone has ESP. This is easier to understand when you think of action, thoughts, and emotions as energetic transmissions. Just like talking and listening, touching and feeling, you send and receive these transmissions with your "extra" senses all the time. As you become familiar with the signals, you'll begin to trust and rely on intuition as another way to gather information. Each time you notice and follow your inner senses, your intuitive perception becomes stronger. When your intuition proves accurate and helpful, it gets validated. When you're totally off track, it will help you listen more carefully. It makes sense to include this inner sensitivity as another way of knowing. Although nobody really understands how this works, it's your personal experience that makes it real and believable. Over time, perception that was previously deemed paranormal or extrasensory will become part of your normal sensory apparatus. Someday, science will be able to tell us how and why.

Intuition Practicum

Honing your intuitive skills means listening to your inner senses and giving them some gravitas. You may feel uncertain and a bit foolish at first. After all, exploring the unknown requires you to take a risk and leave the comfort zone. Because this is new territory and the scientific data is incomplete, you'll need to trust your body, value your experience, and live outside the box. Make no mistake—intuition is an essential component of your body wisdom. When Kim was walking his dog, he didn't question the sequence of events with his mind; his intuitive body just moved into action. Each time you receive, believe, and act on information coming from your inner knowing, the intuition circuitry gets stronger. If your intuition proves trustworthy, give credit where it's due. This is a sign of both security and maturity.

❋ Try This: Let Your Body Choose

If you've never thought of yourself as being intuitive, how can you connect with your inner senses and experience some of this ESP? Just like anything new and strange, you'll need to take a leap of faith. Why not start with something simple like a basic either/or choice? Set out to have some fun, and keep your approach and expectation light and playful. Here's how:

Give yourself a simple wardrobe choice. As you stand in front of two possible options, close your eyes, and let your *body* decide whether to pick up the one on the right or the left. Your choice is not about what you wore yesterday, the weather, or anything your mind already knows. This is about your arm/hand/gut knowing. Don't be surprised if it's hard let go of your visual/mental calculations and trust your body. Just feel which outfit is easy to move toward. Even if you give up and grab the red socks or floral scarf, how do you know it isn't intuition at work? Take a chance on your wardrobe today and see what happens.

You can use this technique to help you with any either/or decision (restaurant, movie, food, and so on). When you place the options side by side, which one does your *body* feel drawn to? For instance, pay attention if you feel an impulse to move, see the right opening, hear the answer, sense an emotional impression, or feel a certainty in your gut. Make the choice without using your eyes, ears, or mind.

Mike. As an abstract artist, Mike had a lot of leeway to follow his inner knowing. Experimenting with trial and error, he observed that his best work happened when he got out of his mind and into his body. His intuition was his best muse. Roadblocks developed when he tried to think about what color to use, how to balance the composition, or where to go. He also noticed that his paintings never had the same charm, magic, or appeal when his mind was in control. All one had to do was look at the canvas; it was easy to tell if Mike's heart was in it. Perhaps all creative people (artists, poets, performers, designers, inventors) get their inspiration through the intuition channel.

✾ Try This: Fork in the Road

The next time you need to decide where to put your energy, which job to take, or what decision to make, ask your intuition to weigh in. Once your mind has mulled over the particulars, close your eyes and imagine you're standing at a fork in the road. Assign each possibility its own direction, take a moment to check in with your inner senses, and let your body choose. Does your personal space expand when you approach one and constrict when you move toward the other? Do your legs and feet feel drawn to one road? Does your inner vision light up with vivid color or seem dull and flat? Is one way enlivened by birdsong or sweet music while the other is deadly silent? Which road or option seems to be easy, unimpeded, and beckoning? Chances are if you follow your intuition, you'll make the right choice.

Clay. Clay was torn between spending the evening at a sports bar with friends and participating in an online seminar. Since he couldn't make up his mind, he decided to try the fork in the road technique. At first he felt silly; communicating with his body as if it were a separate intelligence was definitely bizarre. Out of the blue, he heard a voice say, "Trust your heart." As strange as it may sound, when Clay put his hand on his chest, he felt his chest tighten slightly when he imagined the seminar. He took the feeling as a sign that he should go to the sports bar, even though his mind said it was a frivolous and unproductive choice. As it happened, he met an important new contact that night and later heard the seminar was disappointing. Could his intuition have known all along?

Ben. *Several years ago, Ben was ready to pursue his lifelong dream of selling his home, buying a yacht, and sailing for a bit. He'd retired, fixed up his house, and his realtor had sent in the MLS listing … but something wasn't right. As he sat on his porch and imagined moving forward with his plan, his body felt heavy and dull. Although he'd made up his mind, his body didn't want to move forward. This inner dilemma churned up some doubt, so Ben put his plan on hold for a bit. It soon became clear how helpful his intuition had been. Over the next few months, delaying the real estate deal became a shrewd choice indeed, as the housing market soared. Now, he had an extra $100,000 and it was easy to imagine climbing on board.*

What if you listened to your inner senses for all important decisions? As your intuition proves its reliability on the small stuff, hopefully you'll feel more confident when the big stuff comes along. The next time you come to a fork in the road of life and want to know the right timing, right job, right city, right partnership, or right decision, invite your intuitive body to participate. Once your mind learns to share the power and trust the outcome, it'll welcome the input.

❀ Try This: Turn On Your I-Channel

For reliable guidance any time, turn on the I-channel and go to the source that represents all of your personal interests. As a mentor of mine once said, "The resource is there, you'd be a fool not to use it!" Here's how to proceed: Pose a specific or general question that has to do with your personal good. Then sit quietly and ask the space within, "What do I need to know? What are my assets/challenges? Who are my allies? What are the drawbacks? What are the benefits? What's the biggest picture for the greatest good?" Take your time and proceed systematically. Invite your cognitive mind to step aside, turn on your I-channel and wait for a feeling, insight, phrase, face, sensation, or scenario. Release any physical or mental tension around each question and let the answer float to the surface from deep inside. Be sure to write down your extrasensory response and assess its efficacy in real life. For a while your rational mind might harbor some doubt and forget to credit the source of your brilliance. When you become adept, you'll learn to value the broadcast from your I-channel.

Intuitive knowing can come to you instantaneously, like a flash of insight. And just as often, it can take some time as your subliminal process mulls things over. Once you've posed the question, your inner senses will keep working on it, whether it takes five seconds, five minutes, or five days. Go on with your everyday life, keep the I-channel open, and expect a response. Like an internet search engine, your intuition has a vast data bank of resources, memory, and experience. Don't be surprised if your answer pops up as a metaphor or symbol. Look for a random image, a snippet of poetry, an old adage, a phrase of a song, a dream, or even a random conversation overheard in the marketplace. As you'll discover, your intuition connection has a taproot deep in your imaginative body.

Good intuition is an incredible asset. The more you use it in real time/real life, the less extraordinary and more natural it feels. Once your intuitive connection is online and ready to go, you'll make better decisions, feel more secure, trust your judgment, be less anxious, and respond to situations more appropriately. Sounds pretty amazing, doesn't it? After a while, you'll come to rely on your ESP as much as you do regular perception.

❋ Explore: Cognitive versus Intuitive

One of the assignments for your intuition practicum is to pay attention to what your mind is up to. What do you think about all of this? Can experience change your mind? Your assumptions, self-talk, resistance, emotions, and insights will tell you a lot about how your mind is set. To shake things up a bit, let your intuitive intelligence be the boss for a while. Invite your mind to drop back and be the curious observer. Notice what happens and what happens next. Does intuition add a helpful dimension to your decision-making? Do your inner senses enhance your artful living? Did your inner knowing spring any surprises or change your idea about the breadth and depth of perception? What insights and new understanding have you gleaned from all of the exercises in this practicum? Put your thoughts and experiences down in your journal. As you write, see if your hand, heart, or inner knowing wants to write more and do it. Letting your hand rather than your mind push the pen is called *automatic writing* and is another way to access your intuitive knowing.

Once you have a rudimentary idea of how it functions, why not put your intuition to work and do some personal research? This entails exploring for your own satisfaction rather than taking exact measurements and setting up double-blind studies. It means having some unusual adventures and collecting some interesting anecdotes to tell your friends.

Intuition for Life

Your intuitive body is a great sounding board for good communication and decision-making. It's also a reliable guide for both everyday and extraordinary situations. Listen to your body and it'll tell you whether to go ahead, slow down, or stop. Listen a little deeper and it'll deliver an insight for spot-on choices and timing. Don't worry; your inner knowing is not magical thinking! Magical thinking comes from your mind and can lead you astray. Intuitive thinking is wired to your no-nonsense body. Tune in now and let your intuition become one more facet of your body wisdom.

Intuition for Health

How can your intuition help you get healthy and stay healthy? To have radiant wellness, you need to be responsive to your body's changing needs. Like you explored in the chapter on healing, being aware of your body means being aware of the subtleties of energy, flow, and comfort. If anything is "off," you don't feel "on." In a very real sense, this means responding to a shift in equilibrium before a sore throat, fatigue, or headache shows up. It means choosing the right wellness practitioners and protocols. When your health situation is a little more complicated and returning to balance a little more challenging, trusting your intuition isn't just helpful—it's crucial. Being health-wise means letting your intuitive intelligence join your cognitive intelligence to evaluate what's going on and who or what will help.

> *Leticia.* *Leticia was a high-level, functioning intuitive. It was simply second nature for her to include her intuitive body in any choice or decision. Yet when she faced a serious health issue, she trusted everyone except herself. The source of the problem was eluding her professional team, causing her to panic. One night, she dreamed she was scared and alone in a house where she couldn't turn on the lights. Thinking about her dream the next morning, Leticia got the insight that her body was the house and her problem was the wiring. Following this intuitive tip, she went to see a neurologist who deter-*

mined that the wide range of seemingly disparate symptoms was caused by a tumor. Leticia's inner knowing sent a message, and fortunately she listened.

Don't be shy about bringing your intuition with you to your health care provider. A good health professional wants to know what *you* know about your body. If yours doesn't, maybe you need to look around.

> **Harriet.** *When Harriet took a fall and ruptured two discs, she experienced pain and disability that couldn't be overlooked. She'd been self-sufficient all her life but now had to ask for help. She'd often ignored her body in the past but now was stopped in her tracks, needing to hear her intuitive body and see the bigger picture. It soon became clear that this particular injury at this particular time was the perfect setup for some long-overdue healing, both physical and emotional. Being incapacitated meant Harriet had a lot of time to review her life. Being in pain meant she had a lot of reasons to cry and grieve. And needing other people meant she had to change her attitude and learn to receive. Once she expanded her perspective, it dawned on her that healing wasn't just about the body—it was about healing her whole person so she could shift gears and align with a deeper truth.*

Intuition for Love

Developing your intuition helps you connect with other people. Because intuition naturally resonates with authenticity (yours and theirs), it's a resource for honesty in any situation. When it comes to love, however, your intuitive alignment is key for accurate perception, timing, and communication. Anytime you need to negotiate the interactive complexities of two people in one relationship, your ability to read nonverbal signals, respond appropriately, have good boundaries, and be insightful comes in handy. Being intimate is much easier when you know and trust your intuitive body.

> **Mac.** *Mac met someone who could be "the one." This new guy had all the essential attributes and seemed attracted to him as well. Having loved many times and lost, Mac felt cautious and distrusted his love choices. Rather than listen to his lustful body, this time he chose to listen to his intuitive body, which meant getting close before getting intimate. Slowing down meant he could hear, feel, and see things with*

more perspective. His own sense of space helped him keep good boundaries and relate to another whole person rather than his own fantasy. Following his intuition and taking the time for love helped Mac trust and respect himself as well as his partner. This was an auspicious beginning for a successful love relationship.

Truthfully, when it comes to love, your mind might not know what's best for you. Your mind can concoct all kinds of fantasies and arguments that crumble under the scrutiny of intuition. Your intuitive body doesn't lie. Tune in and you'll know if your inner feelings are lined up with what's happening. Pay attention and you'll know when to move toward a relationship, when to move away, and when it's time to move on. Listen and you'll know how to communicate. Relax and take your time. Be authentic with yourself and your partner as you build trust, respect, and intimacy. Let your intuition expand the scope of love from "I" to "we."

Krista. One more time, Krista brought up a perennially unresolved issue with her partner. As they circled this old conflict, she didn't feel anger or sorrow… she just felt surreal. It was as if both of them had vacated the premises and their words were disembodied. At this impasse, her inner knowing made it clear that no one was onboard to make the changes necessary. Without blame or shame, the relationship had simply run its course and it was time to move on. Sharing her insight created the most graceful, powerful, and irrefutable way to end the relationship.

Listen in before you speak up. Whenever you have feelings or issues you want to share, run it by your body first. If your throat tightens, your ears buzz, or your eyesight gets fuzzy, maybe this is not the time or place. If the words just seem to flow, you're on the right track. Let your intuition be a part of the conversation. Are you getting through? What feelings are present? Is there an underlying agenda or issue that needs to be addressed? Your comfort level will let you know if:

- You're making a positive impression
- You're being received with love and respect
- You've stayed too long or gone too far

Alyssa. *Alyssa and her current beau had a rough evening. Both of them had their feelings hurt over a seemingly silly misunderstanding. The next day, they texted from work repeatedly to resolve the problem but it just seemed to get worse. Wanting to find a way to shift the focus from "you said/I said," Alyssa took her lunch break to sit quietly and let her intuitive body show her the root of the problem. As she tuned in, she felt a familiar set of her jaw that reminded her of endless power struggles with her father. Separating the past from the present was a way to see beyond the particulars of the argument and focus on the emotional healing it offered. When the timing felt right, she invited her boyfriend to dinner and shared her insight and personal process. Alyssa's honesty and integrity deepened the intimacy of the relationship.*

If you've lived and loved, chances are you've encountered extrasensory input at one time or another. You think of someone and they call; you say something and they exclaim, "I was just thinking about that!" You *know* if someone is being truthful or not. You *feel* the nonverbal communication and *see* the emotional subtext. Intimacy implies an intuitive connection. Your regular senses and cognitive mind give you a lot of information, but your inner senses give you the inside scoop.

Intuition for Social Success

Being intuitive means being successful in any social situation. It's easy to be an effective communicator when you can recognize nonverbal signals and respond appropriately. It's easy to establish trust and receptivity when you're comfortable, authentic, and have good boundaries. Listening with your inner senses sharpens your receptors and improves your ability to connect (or disconnect). Because intuition is hardwired to emotional intelligence, it increases your ability to perceive and address unexpressed feelings or unspoken agendas. When you see where a conversation is going and have a sense where it's coming from, you have the information to be graceful and inclusive. This is important for problem-solving as well as conflict resolution. Being insightful is one attribute of a highly functioning, social person.

Alfred. *Alfred was having a conversation with his new brother-in-law at Thanksgiving dinner. When the topic shifted from sports to politics, Alfred felt his throat tighten. This was a clear signal from his intuitive body that he couldn't speak freely.*

When he strategically changed the course of the conversation to the weather, his tension relaxed and the interaction stayed congenial. After all, this wasn't about being right or making a point, this was about creating a successful relationship. Rather than fan the flames of something potentially contentious, Alfred chose to keep the conversation civil and gracious. Family gatherings would probably be more successful if everyone arrived with their emotional intelligence and intuitive sensibility.

Cherie. *Since it was her turn to host the book group, Cherie got to pick the book. A month later, when the ladies got together to discuss the book, Cherie noticed some discord in her otherwise serene living room. When the group had settled in, rather than override her intuition, she looked around and said, "So, what's up?" Because she was so present and open, Cherie created a safe container to talk about the emotional undercurrent. It was soon revealed that the theme of the book, losing a child, was also a member's personal story. The ensuing discussion allowed each person to talk about loss and grief at a very personal level. As a result, the bond between the women deepened and everyone went home feeling good. Cherie had turned a potential social disaster into a successful evening of intimacy and healing.*

Intuition for Business

Being intuitive gives you the foresight to anticipate consequences and find solutions. It also enhances your communication and managerial skills. When you use your intuitive intelligence you can hear the unspoken agendas and see the hidden landmines. You can decipher the problems as well as the potentials in any business situation. Over time, your associates will recognize your business acumen (deal skills) as well as your authenticity and trustworthiness. In the business world, sensitivity is often discouraged and seen as a negative trait. But being sensitive doesn't mean being emotional. Bring your intuition to work with you for the "insight edge" in any business endeavor.

Theresa. *A new client sat in Theresa's therapy office, and the air was charged with anxious energy. Being sensitive to the situation, Theresa knew that first and foremost, she'd need to create an environment of trust and safety. She did this by soliciting her client's comfort and making some small talk before asking anything personal. By demonstrating her sensitivity, Theresa communicated her trustworthiness. Theresa's intuitive* timing was an essential prerequisite for a therapeutic relationship. As such, it ensured the success of the session and set the tone for future healing.

Peter. At the monthly board meeting, Peter brought up an important project for discussion. Though everyone in the room seemed supportive, Peter's stomach wouldn't relax—his gut feeling told him that something wasn't right. Scanning the room for nonverbal communication, he made a note that one of the principals was literally holding back with arms crossed and eyes lowered. Rather than be confrontational and address her directly, Peter said he wondered if anyone had any insights to share about the project. At this opening, the hesitant person spoke up and expressed her reservation about one of the investors. Later, when the company did a little further research, it was clear that the investor was indeed overextended and unlikely to follow through as promised. Because he interpreted his colleague's resistance as information rather than personal opposition, Peter could stay open to vital information he might have missed otherwise. In the process, he'd trusted his intuition and hers.

Chuck. Chuck took a colleague out to lunch to talk about collaborating on a production. Each time he started to pitch his idea, he got interrupted—the waiter arrived, he got a phone call, and a friend stopped by the table to say hi. Rather than push against the resistance, Chuck spent the time talking about this and that and building general goodwill. On the drive home, an old Louis Armstrong song popped into his head. Wondering what the lyrics to "Let's Call the Whole Thing Off" might mean, Chuck realized his intuition was sending him a message. It was telling him to find a different partner who'd be more in sync with his vision and goals. Chuck avoided an awkward mistake and got on track for success when he listened to intuition.

Ming. Ming is a successful designer in large part because she follows her artistic intuition. Recently she was doing a high-end job and wanted something tropical and unique to anchor the focus in her client's living room. She had the color scheme and the furniture placement but hadn't gotten the go ahead for the wall treatment. Even though the architect and builder were impatient, Ming took the night to sleep on it. The next morning, her intuition gave her the standard 4:00 am wake-up call with the image of a painting she'd seen recently at MoMA. Using this as an inspiration for a wall mural would work perfectly! It was as if her "inner artist" had known all along and just needed an avenue to communicate.

Intuition for Changing Times

Developing your intuition helps you negotiate the rocky waters of uncertain and turbulent times. There has been more change in the past fifty years than at any other time in history, and it seems the pace isn't slowing any time soon. Being intuitive helps you adapt to these changing times. Instead of getting caught up in a spin of resistance or confusion, listening to your deep knowing and seeing the big picture helps you stay resilient, responsive, and calm. Heed your intuitive intelligence when making crucial decisions and building reliable relationships. Listen to your intuitive sensibilities if you want to avoid discord, anticipate danger, and respond effectively to the world at large. When the pace of change speeds up, your intuitive connection makes the difference between feeling empowered and feeling overwhelmed.

> *Sue. Often solutions to problems and personal insights come to Sue when she's dancing. Anytime Sue needs guidance or insight, she puts on music and dances until the a-ha! moment arrives. Typically, as her body begins to move, her mind lets go and a flash of insight simply appears. She trusts her dancing intuition to solve problems, receive guidance, and do personal healing. And, whenever she feels unhappy or uncertain, she sets aside some time to dance and connect with the rhythms of the cosmos. Doing so always gives her comfort, security, and a little peek at the big picture.*

To some people, these examples might border on the far-out world of psychic phenomena. To others, they may be everyday experiences. When your intuition connection is plugged in, there's nothing mystical or unusual about receiving information from your inner senses. It's simply a matter of tuning in and paying attention to the feedback coming from your own body.

Intuition for the Spiritual Journey

Being an intuitive person ultimately means being able to listen to both your inner self and your higher self. Once your intuition gets tested and proved worthy in real life, being intuitive will become a new normal. Afterward, extrasensory perception will simply be another way to gather information. As you go through life and encounter the inevitable unknowns, whys, and wherefores, it'll be reassuring to know that your intuition isn't baffled by the mysterious or unknown. It's an existential comfort to your linear, logical mind when intuition opens the door to spiritual understanding. What if, in the course of your busy life, you remembered to pause and see the light, hear a whisper of grandmother's wisdom, and feel aligned with the universe? What if you took the time to be quiet and marvel in wonder without having to analyze or control? Feeling a personal connection to the beyond is your intuitive portal to your spiritual self.

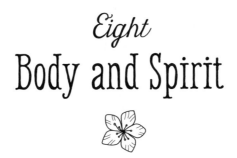

Eight
Body and Spirit

An intimate relationship with your conscious body opens the door to spirit. As you've already discovered, being in the moment, emptying your mind, and expanding your awareness is facilitated when you're in tune with your body. Tuning in to your body can also be a way to approach the seemingly ethereal world of things bigger and beyond your small self. Rather than something intangible, what if spirit was as close as your breath or your feet touching the ground? What if being spiritual was a normal, ordinary function of being alive?

In so many ways, from the very beginning, spirit has been a part of your physical life. As you become more body-wise, the presence of this other dimension just becomes more apparent. Have you noticed that things seem to work out better when you listen to your body's inner knowing? When you follow intuition, do you benefit from seemingly random coincidences and unexpected opportunities? When you feel grateful, do you also feel graceful? This is how spirit shows up in your everyday life. Whenever you experience an insight, synchronicity, or the "peace which surpasses all understanding," giving credit to a spiritual dimension changes the way you see things. Making the body-spirit connection changes how you walk in the world, yet making the body-spirit connection can be difficult if your mind isn't on board.

Open Your Mind

For the purposes here, let's say that "spirit" represents the part of your physical experience that goes beyond dense blood-and-guts reality to include the expansive experience of being alive and connected to a greater mystery. In order to understand and embrace your body's relationship with a larger whole, you may need to let go of preconceived ideas and shift perspective a bit. When you feel connected to something bigger and more complete, it doesn't matter whether it's spirit or life force or higher power.

Try This: Find Your Terms

You've had lots of opportunities in this book to stretch your mind and see things from a different perspective. In order to consider the more ephemeral aspects of life in your body, you need to find the terms that work for you. To take a fresh look, put aside what your mind knows about religion or philosophy and go right to your personal experience. What simple term could you use to describe the part of you that feels loving compassion and connection to something bigger than your small self? How could you speak about inexplicable coincidences and a sense of divine guidance in your life? As you read this chapter, if the words *spirit* or *spiritual* don't work for you, simply replace them with ones that do. Don't let semantics get in the way of expanding your understanding of body and spirit.

Open Your Body

From a physical perspective, the spiritual dimension is focused through your external and internal sense of space. This is the kinesthetic sense that you learned about at the beginning of this book. You open your body to spirit whenever you feel more spacious and less dense. This can happen simply by closing your eyes and feeling expansive beyond your skin. It can also happen when you let go of tension and you sense your muscle mass lightening. Developing your kinesthetic sense is a vital part of being body wise. Having a good sense of space helps you breathe easier, dissipate anxiety, and relieve pain. It's also required for good intimacy and intuition. When you have a good sense of space, it opens the door to a sense of spirit. The French philosopher Pierre Teilhard de

Chardin stated, "We are not human beings having a spiritual experience. We are spiritual beings having a human experience."[27]

A good time to experience this wisdom is at either end of your sleep cycle. Before and after sleep when your cognitive mind is lingering in soft awareness, your sense of self can expand to include spirit space. In this numinous state, you can connect body and spirit simply by breathing. Using breath to feel a connection to something beyond the mundane is a century-old practice used by the Greeks (*pneuma*), Christians (holy spirit), and the Hindus (*prana*). You've already learned how to use your breath to quiet the mind, de-stress the psyche, and connect with others. Hopefully, these experiences have helped you move beyond the delusion of separateness and feel moments of peace and connection. Now it's time to follow your breathing body to find spirit. After all, *spiritu* is the Latin root for both "breath" and "spirit."

❀ Try This: Breathing in Spirit Space

Set yourself up for a few moments of focused quiet time. Close your eyes and tune in to your body. Relax your shoulders and soften your belly. Let the gentle, flowing rhythm of breath expand beyond your belly into the rest of your inner space (bones, skin, muscles, organs, soft tissues, vessels, and fibers). Without any additional effort, feel the gentle undulations spread out further to include the space around your body. Breathe in this expansive, inclusive way until the boundary between inner and outer seems to disappear. Could it be that your own breath, moving just as it was designed to move, connects you energetically with the space around you? Feel the motion of filling/emptying and imagine that the prime mover is spirit rather than body. Drop into the possibility as you pause just a bit at the end of your inhale to feel how your breath seems to flow out all on its own. Pause again at the end of your exhale and notice the air return to your lungs without any effort.

You can explore the expansive feeling of breathing in the most ordinary places. The next time you're waiting for an appointment or for your computer to boot up, take a moment to breathe in spirit space. Do it before you go to sleep tonight and feel how

....

27 *Brainyquote.com*, s.v. "Pierre Teilhard de Chardin," accessed 2017. www.brainyquote.com /quotes.p.pierreteil160888.

your expanded sense of self quiets mind and body. Use it to focus before a meal or find a calm reference point when you're anxious or out of sorts. Breathing in spirit space makes any communication more focused and personal. Tune in and this space deepens your experience of walking in nature, listening to music, or enjoying a work of art. Remember: any place at any time, spirit is just a breath away.

✾ Try This: Feel the Wonder

Your sense of space connects the inner to the outer so you feel at one with the moment and the world around. Your other senses are also on board to help you connect in spiritual ways. If you slow down the pace and dial in your awareness, you can tune out your chattering mind and tune in to spirit. It's easy to include some wonder even as you go about your everyday routines. All you have to do is expand your perception to include:

- The sound of birds in nearby trees, the wind in the chimes, or the rhythmic ebb and flow of the sea

- The air moving across your skin or the sun's warm rays on your arm

- The gentle fragrance of a garden or the rich dampness of the earth

- The dancing light on a wall or the swirling patterns of clouds

As you notice the presence of the world around you, feel your connection to it all. You are a part of this planetary mix and, as such, a part of something bigger and greater than your small self. Suspend your idea of separation and be at one with the extraordinary miracle of life.

Spirit Sense

Feeling a part of something larger is not just a philosophical construct or a random experience. Your wise body is *the* gateway to the expansive world of spirit. What if you could develop an extrasensory faculty—a kind of spirit sensibility? What if perceiving the world through this spirit sense gave the most mundane activities another dimension? And, in this new dimension, it was normal to feel intimately alive and intuitively awake in each micromoment? Just like focusing your eyes to see something sharply or your ears to hear the innuendos, when you bring your attention to your spirit sense, time automatically slows down and space opens up. Whether you're driving on the freeway, planting the spring garden, negotiating a tricky business deal, or casually lunching with friends, your spirit sensibility changes the picture. With just a slight shift of perception, you become a spiritual being having a human experience.

✱ Try This: Get in the Spirit

When you're in the spirit of things, even the routines of your everyday life feel special and inspired. Over the next few days, pause now and again to get aligned with spirit. When you brush your teeth, work out on the treadmill, or walk the dog, let your awareness expand beyond the task (and the mind chatter) to notice the quality of light, the sounds of nature, and your connection to it all. Does this change the way you feel in the moment? When you're solving a problem, interacting with a colleague, or relating to a loved one, let your sense of self expand to include the greater good. Does this give you a broader perspective and deeper insight? Any time you change your orientation from little/singular to big/plural, you get in the spirit of things.

Using your spirit sensibility in any situation changes the equation and changes the outcome. Try it out. If you're dealing with a health issue, a relationship conflict, or an unexpected inconvenience, expand your awareness to include spirit. Challenge your mind to step aside and let your decisions, actions, and interactions originate from your body's sense of oneness with all there is. Can you feel your tension soften? Can you feel your perspective expand? Is there access to more insight and new solutions? Being in the spirit of things means you're less tied to the problem and more open to the solutions.

Preston. Preston had spent many years seeking spiritual knowledge. With a degree in philosophy, he had followed a guru, lived in an ashram, read multitudes of books, and sat daily in meditation. Unfortunately, his pesky body repeatedly got in the way. If it wasn't lower back pain, it was IBS (irritable bowel syndrome) or buzzing in his ears. He just couldn't get beyond his dense, material body to find the realm of spirit. One day in the midst of a painful episode, Preston stopped trying to rise above his body and all things physical. Instead, he included his noisy body as just another beat in the grand symphony of life. By focusing on the many sounds rather than the singular sound, Preston discovered that the distraction of his body was a mere back-ground murmur. Perhaps being spiritual didn't mean leaving his body behind after all. This shift in perspective was a spiritual epiphany.

You don't need to spend years and years searching or put yourself in extreme circumstances to encounter spirit. It is a part of being alive and around you all of the time. In order to tune in, you might need to let go of some preconceived ideas, broaden your perspective, and trust your body. Even if you suspect you're missing something essential and dedicate yourself to the task, finding your spirit sense may still seem exclusive and elusive. You'll be pleased to know that walking on the beach or sitting with your cat are good ways to develop spirit sensibility. Invite spirit in and the most ordinary moment can become extraordinary. Following are some tried and true ways to develop your spirit sense.

Walking Meditation

You are either in the flow or not in the flow when you're walking. This is a body-spirit thing. If you're taking a walk and thinking about this or that, you are *not* in the moment, not in the spirit of things. You are in your mind and in your thoughts—somewhere else. You are in your emotions, in your story, and somewhere else. The very simple act of walking consciously is a time-honored technique to develop awareness. Being aware of your body in action not only quiets the mind and the emotions, it brings you into the spirit of the moment. Practicing a walking meditation is an easy way to bring your body, mind, and spirit into alignment.

❀ Try This: Walking Meditation

Find a place to walk that is flat and clear of obstacles. Stand for a few moments with your full awareness on your body. Feel your feet on the ground. Let your mind focus on your standing balance. Then shift your whole body slightly forward to initiate the momentum for walking. As you take each step, notice how each foot moves through a unique range of motion and each leg swings in its own design. Notice how the motion includes the rest of your body (pelvis, back, shoulders, neck, and head). As your arms and legs swing naturally, let your body synchronize with this basic movement. Imagine that you are walking as effortlessly as possible. Continue walking in this manner, letting your eyes rest on the horizon and your muscle intelligence lead the way. Notice if there is any holding or bracing and let it go with the flow. Observe how you disconnect from the step/swing action when your thinking mind takes over. Return to the simple, fluid motion of your anatomy every time your mind wanders. This basic walking meditation is a great way to develop your spirit sense.

Will. Will stood on a stretch of the beach for a few moments before he began walking. As he scanned through his body, he noticed that everything felt relaxed except his clenched hands. He let his hands soften and began with the first slow small step, followed by the next. A couple of minutes into his walking meditation, Will became aware that his hands were tense again. At first, he thought this was a random habit but then he realized that every time his mind drifted away from the simple act of walking (heel to toe, leg to leg), his hands clenched. This led to a simple epiphany—it was impossible to be focused on his thoughts and moving body at the same time. If he kept his awareness in his loose hands, it helped him stay in the flow and stay in the moment.

Go into Nature

Throughout the ages, seekers have gone into the wilderness to find a deeper connection, a greater wisdom. Although an aesthetic retreat on a solitary mountain might be a profound experience, you don't have to go on a vision quest or sit in a cave to develop your spirit sense. Anytime, anywhere you diminish the distraction of the human world and align with the natural world creates a bridge to a greater, deeper wisdom. To develop your spirit sense in nature, get out of your house and into the world of plants and animals, rocks, and clouds. Linger there; ask a question; open yourself to guidance. Go natural and invite some insight and oversight from the realm of spirit.

❋ Try This: Communing with Nature

Getting away from the cacophony of the human-centered, high tech world is a good way to tune in to the more subtle vibrations of spirit. To actually get up close and commune with nature, you'll also need a degree of privacy so you don't feel foolish and minimal distraction so you stay focused. Sit quietly and close your eyes. Focus on the immediacy of the moment and let the issues, dramas, schedules, and responsibilities of your human world drift away. Tune in to the essence, tempo, and space around you. Can you sense color, energy vibration, or the presence of spirit? Does your bit of nature seem to be flowing or pulsing, steady or still? Invite your body to slow down to "nature time," measured in day/night, seasons, and eons. Let yourself be a part of the innate balance and synchrony of this moment. Feel how your presence and life force are an integral part of this space. When you develop some spirit sense in nature, it might feel as if your sense of separateness is just an illusion. Once you return to the mostly peopled world, why not let spirit come with you?

Tracy. Tracy bought a cottage in the Berkshires to rest and rejuvenate. For the first few months, her habitual busyness powered through each weekend and the pace of the country felt just as hectic as city life. As the novelty eventually wore off, nature won out. Tracy began to notice a new sensitivity to the comings and goings of bird and beast; the gurgling sound of the stream out back; the smells of an oncoming storm or a change of season. As her mind quieted, the natural world got louder. For Tracy, leaving the intensity of the city gave her a chance to feel her essence and replenish her creativity. And what a delight to feel her body downshift to "country time" the minute she crossed the Henry Hudson Bridge!

Susannah. Susannah discovered that her "spirit sight" improved when she took vision out of the picture. In her poetic words, "When I take a walk, I close my eyes so I can sense my feet on the ground, feel the breeze, and catch the scent in the air from the wild grasses. I often put my hands out on either side to touch tall flowers, branches or the silky feel of the high grasses. With my eyes closed, it's as if the soft breeze flows through me and I can feel the day's beginning stir the air with the fragrance of new-morning dampness and the sea." Anytime things are pressing on her, Susannah takes a walk to feel connected to spirit and lighten up. Being in nature's cathedral is a vital part of her spiritual practice.

Kate. Being a money manager and scientifically oriented, it seems improbable that Kate would have a relationship with a tree. But whenever Kate wants input from spirit, she hikes a certain mountain trail to seek the counsel of a particular tree. Her first encounter with this source of wisdom happened quite by accident. One day, while walking along and mulling over a particular issue, the guidance she needed seemed to come out of the blue from a particular oak. Wondering if this was just her imagination, she brought another problem to the tree on her next hike and it happened again! Not only has this tree's wisdom been helpful, it has changed her idea about the sentient connection of all life. As Kate explained it, "My tree has lived so many more years than I have, seen the comings and goings of lots of human drama, and knows about balance right down to its roots."

Relating to Animals

Being around animals is another way to develop your spirit sense and feel connected to all life. If you've had a relationship with a pet, you probably learned the basic Buddhist tenet of being present and loving unconditionally. Just touching an animal can make the trauma-drama of the news cycle, demands of your schedule, and urgency of ambition seem to fade away. Like communing with nature, when you spend sweet, simple time with an animal, you can get beyond your self-centered orientation to align with the subtle essence of spirit.

> **Christine.** *Christine calls her cat's calming presence "the healing paws (pause)." Anytime she feels upset, spacey, or wired she knows holding her cat in her lap will help her shift gears, quiet her mind, and find her spirit center. There's something about relating to animals that creates a link to the earth and basic rhythms of life. Being in cat space has taught Christine to empty her mind, open her heart, and feel connected. In this way, her cat is one of her spiritual teachers.*

❀ Try This: Listen to the Animals

The next time you're in the presence of an animal see if you can downshift to the pace and simplicity of animal time. After all, you're an animal too. Instead of speeding along on the trajectory of your thoughts, let your breath measure the cadence. See if you can slow down and quiet your heart enough to create a space for relationship. Linger for as long as you can in animal time and open your mind to learn something new. Dr. Dolittle aside, it might surprise you to discover a deeper understanding and a spiritual kinship with the animal kingdom around you.

Leo. Leo's mom and dad took him with some regularity to Little Farm to feed the cows and goats. At first he was totally terrified of the big, strange beasts and their eager mouths. But he was intrigued and kept asking to go back. At each visit, his parents encouraged him to pay attention, take it slowly, and trust his body. It wasn't long before Leo could offer a stick of celery to the goats and cows with boldness and confidence. Along with his growing comfort with animals, Leo seemed to be more grounded and comfortable with himself. Tuning in to the animal channel helped his parents slow down, calm down, and feel some spirit as well.

Gifted dog and horse trainers use their spirit sense to tune in to the animal channel. To do this, they neutralize any mental and emotional disturbance and align with the tempo of breath. Any time you want to relate to animals, even from afar, you'll have more success if you get out of your small thinking mind and into your big sense of spirit. My friend Guerdon free-dives and explores his spirit sense in the sea. When he encounters a fish, he quiets his mind and simply hangs out as long as he can. And, when Guerdon spends time in this way with the fish, he returns to land with a profound sense of spiritual contentment. My friend Kathleen says, "Being with animals is about losing all ego and listening to the wisdom of another species. This is a direct link with spirit and requires an open heart and quiet mind." For all of these people, being with animals helps them get in touch with something bigger than their small self.

Spiritual Sex

Everyone knows you can have good sex and bad sex, but *spiritual* sex? Just like everywhere else in your life, when you open your experience to include spirit, being sexual can be a bridge from your small self to your big self and the world beyond. Could this be the difference between satisfaction and ecstasy? If you're stuck in the physical dimension, it's easy for your spirit sense to get sidelined by distractions of performance, fantasy, and body mechanics. With your mind and body taking up so much space, spiritual intimacy is held at bay. Here's how to get your body *and* spirit aligned for spiritual intimacy:

- Approach sex as an expression of your connection to spirit

- Focus 100 percent on the physical—no tension, no time line, and no agenda

- Include the sacred space of your body, your partner's body, and beyond

- Trust your body's innate knowledge and let it lead the way

- Stay in the moment with each inhale and exhale

- Be centered in body-spirit consciousness as intensity builds

- Linger in the transcendent feeling of oneness

Throughout this book you've learned about the importance of being awake and aware. Spiritual sex is an opportunity to be awake and aware with someone else, let the two become one, and something more.

Alan. The routine of sex had lost its fascination for Alan. Although it was physically satisfying, he was mentally and spiritually bored. Recently, he turned this around when he brought his Buddhist practice into the bedroom. Rather than veering off in his usual fantasy scenario, Alan adapted his mindfulness techniques and stayed present. As he explained, "When I'm connected to my body and the moment, it changes the way my body moves and my hands touch. My breathing and desire become something shared with my partner instead of a solo experience. If my mind wanders, I bring it back to my body and its way of expressing divine love." For Alan, including spirit was the key to renewing his passion.

Throughout time, seekers have explored ways to transform sexual energy into spiritual energy. Because it's such a compelling, transformative experience, your sexuality can be a powerful way to connect to spirit. When you bring body and spirit into the same picture, you're opening the door to one of life's great sacred mysteries—we are all one, with all life.

Get Aligned

In a very physical sense, your body and spirit have a natural alignment. To get a feel for this, sit or lie down and get comfortable. Visualize an invisible cord linking the space above your head to your heart, your pelvis, legs, feet, and the space below your feet in a direct line. This is your central channel. Survey the pipeline of this channel and use your breath to dislodge and open any places that are blocked or crowded. Once it clears, linger in this place of spirit alignment and let your breath be the only measure of time. Can you feel the lightness of air move through your bones, organs, and soft tissues? Do you feel more and more at one (inside and outside) with spirit space? In this place of both emptiness and connection, you'll probably feel more kinship with your spirit body and less affinity for your material body. This is the natural domain of spirit.

Your body's spiritual alignment comes in handy anytime you need reassurance or seek guidance from a higher source. But, in times of change and challenge, knowing how to get and stay aligned is essential. As you know from experience, life is not always smooth sailing; sometimes a storm descends or turbulence throws you off and it's hard to sort it out. At such times, the reliable old adage "this too shall pass" may seem like a hollow promise when everything around you is in turmoil. But if you tune in to your alignment with the heavens above and the earth below through the central channel, it gives you a lifeline that will see you through.

Sam. Following some harsh life lessons, Sam was feeling isolated and small. In the past, he'd just fill his calendar with work, exercise, and distraction to get through. But this strategy was hardly comforting and never satisfying. This time, Sam decided to do it differently and use the situation to find a deeper truth. So, instead of accelerating through, he asked his spirit sense to take the lead. Instead of rushing to get away, he went toward it and felt how his emotional discomfort was blocking his spiritual flow. Instead of focusing on his problems as issues, Sam decided to let them be residue. Bit by bit, chakra by chakra, he was able to clear the debris and open his central channel. One day when he was practicing spiritual alignment, Sam experienced the transcendent feeling of being a sentient body sitting in sentient space. In this place of clarity he realized that spirit would help him move beyond even the most unpleasant situation.

Once you develop a sense of spirit, you perceive things differently. Everyday circumstances give you opportunities to practice your body wisdom. The whole picture changes when you can see clearly, hear guidance, and feel at one with spirit. Instead of being alone and limited, you feel connected and infinite. From the standpoint of your body, this is both grounding and calming. From the standpoint of your mind, it's reassuring and empowering. The simple truth is when body and spirit are plugged in, every turn in the road has the potential to bring you to a place of gracefulness and Grace.

Spirit Sense for Extraordinary Times

Having spirit sense is essential whenever you experience loss, illness, injury, trauma, drama, or mishap. At such times, it can feel as if your body and mind are caught up in an unrelenting storm of panic and confusion. This is actually the result of a physiological strategy designed to help you through overwhelming situations. But if your spirit sense is not part of the equation, this management strategy can create *more* stress and upset. During extraordinary times, you need your big perspective more than ever. When all else is in flux, your connection to spirit helps you trust the process, stay centered, and keep the faith. Here are some specific ways to use some spirit sense when you need it the most.

Injury and Illness

Anytime your body gets stopped in its tracks (from a minor twist of the ankle to life-threatening illness), a spiritual perspective helps you be patient, slow down, and attend to the business of healing. How comforting to let the hurt, fear, and frustration be viewed without judgment in the context of a big picture. How reassuring to feel a semblance of certainty and positive input from a big knowing. How soothing to release the emotional and physical trauma of pain to a big space. Not only does your spirit sense offer you comfort and focus, it's a resource for insight and inspiration from a Big Source.

Having a good connection to spirit is vitally important when healing takes a long time. If your health is compromised for weeks and months, the ordeal can sideline your positive thinking with turmoil, despair, and confusion. When you're in for the long haul, listening to your body's spirit sense may be the key to clarity and reclaiming your power. This is the perfect time to focus on the alignment of your central channel with the source of all healing—spirit. This is the perfect time to expand your spirit space to include a context that is both hopeful and helpful. This is the perfect time to ask your spirit guides for the insight and oversight to help you be patient, manage your doubts and fears, and envision the healing you need. If you can find a deeper, larger meaning, the tedious details of the day-to-day seem to fade a bit. Remember, when you're stuck in the isolation and/or pain of a long-term illness, let spirit give you solace with each breath you take. How comforting to know that spirit accompanies you on your healing journey.

Emotional Trauma

When circumstances send a shock wave through your emotional body, it can be a relief to just be numb for a while. This natural response is the initial way the body-mind copes with trauma. It's as if your body and spirit occupy separate spaces. After a certain interval, in order to heal, your body-spirit needs to realign. If you've experienced this condition, you know about that empty, vacant, dull feeling. If you've been around someone who's suffered emotional trauma, you've observed the "no one's at home" condition. Your body wisdom can help you neutralize emotional trauma and return to full physical presence. When you're ready, use your spirit sense to connect with something bigger than your small self. This will give you the perspective and incentive to begin healing. Invite spirit into the process. Let the breathing and alignment practices you've learned in this chapter be like a prayer that gets repeated over and over again. These are your touchstones for healing. Put your trust in spirit and it will lead you step by step back to body, mind, and spirit harmony.

Mental Illness

From your body's perspective, mental illness affects your energy and energy field much like a chronic health situation. All of the ways that your spirit sense shows up for emotional and physical healing are helpful when your mind needs grounding, balancing, and faith. In addition to seeking professional help, this is the time to reach for something more reliable than your small self. Making a regular practice of getting your body up and moving (exercise, tai chi, dance, yoga) puts your feet on solid ground. Tuning in to the steady cadence of your breathing gives you a familiar reference point, and invoking the support and guidance of spirit cultivates hope. In addition to the physiological benefits of moving and breathing, including the spiritual dimension simply gives you a sense of volition and some peace of mind. In times of crisis, this can be a blessing when all else seems out of control. As a daily practice, including spirit can set the foundation for new behaviors and perspectives.

Spiritual Crisis

Maybe once or twice in a lifetime, you'll find yourself in a spiritual crisis. At such times, everything you know and trust is in upheaval. When your sense of self is questioned and your beliefs are no longer grounded in certitude, it can feel as if your world has fallen apart. If seen from a spiritual perspective, this isn't actually a disaster. Rather, it's an opportunity to grow, re-evaluate, and align with your deepest truth. It's a time to trust the unknown, to move into new realms of discovery. It may seem as if spirit has abandoned you but your spirit sense hasn't. Even in the worst crisis, you can still feel the physical presence of each breath and your body's connection to the earth below, the heavens above. Let your spirit sense lead the way and imagine that each step and each breath you take aligns you with spirit, over and over again. Be patient, await your epiphany, and look for the light at the end of the tunnel. Open yourself to the guidance of your inner and outer senses (such as ESP) and trust that your confusion and despair will be resolved when the crisis subsides.

Anytime you find yourself in extraordinary circumstances, remember spirit. Your spirit sensibility won't just get you through, it'll deepen your understanding of the mystery and change your life. In my clinical practice, I've seen many clients come up against a circumstance that forced them to stop, wake up, pay attention, and change course. Often, before they could heal, they needed to discover, include, and listen to spirit. Sometimes, they had to enlarge their perspective in order to find the key to opening and moving on. What if you have to fall apart in order to come together again? What if you need to walk away from everything familiar in order to find yourself? What if your "dark night of the soul" is the way to an intimate relationship with spirit?

Kim. When Kim found out she had rheumatoid arthritis she felt backed into a corner with nothing to look forward to beyond the diagnosis. She felt overwhelmed by the task ahead, unable to cope and hope. Kim needed to find a way to get bigger than the diagnosis. One day, in despair, Kim remembered her deeper body wisdom and used her sense of space to get bigger than her condition. Curiously, the pain seemed to soften. Like a lifeline, Kim returned day after day to this place that offered such emotional and physical reprieve. Eventually, she had the epiphany that her body and its journey were only part of the story. Once she could see beyond her fear, her fear was no longer crippling. Once she could see beyond her isolation, she began to seek and be grateful for the help she needed. This simple shift in perspective was, indeed, a gift from spirit.

Carlo. *When Carlo's marriage fell apart, it felt as if his whole life disassembled. Nothing felt familiar and the old gambits of blaming, manipulating, and striving no longer worked. He just had to find a way to "deal." As he sat in a stew of emotions, Carlo searched for something familiar to hold onto in a world turned upside down. Although his mind was numb, he could at least feel his feet touch the floor. Using this reference point to ground himself, he heard himself say, "I am here." A few days later, he noticed that he'd synchronized this coping strategy with his breath saying on the inhale "I am" and on the exhale "here." Carlo had stumbled on the perfect body-spirit mantra that helped him feel both centered in his own being and connected to something bigger. Day by day he began to re-establish the simple routines that made his life feel normal again. And when the right relationship came along, he was ready rather than needy.*

Living in Sacred Space

Your body is a bridge to spirit for both everyday and extraordinary times. It's also home base for a spiritual practice. Throughout this book, tuning in to your wise body has helped you expand your awareness, deepen your understanding, and show up for a happy and healthy life. Your wise body can now help you show up for a spiritual life. The truth is, no matter how familiar, satisfied, or comfortable you feel in your body, you haven't really arrived until spirit is in residence. Body and spirit are *not* mutually exclusive. Yet, sometimes, we assume a hierarchy where the spirit part is loftier than the body part. When this happens, spiritual seekers get caught in the trap of judging or resenting the distractions and demands of their body. What if your body was a part of spirit and spirit was a part of your body? Perhaps you should invite your body to be your spiritual guide.

Enders. Enders noticed that his face had a hard time staying neutral when he meditated. He never felt the exact moment when his tongue started pushing and jaw tightened, but this familiar holding pattern snuck in over and over again. One day, instead of letting go, Enders held onto the tension and looked at it without judgment. From this perspective, it was so clear that his tight mouth held an expression of grim disgust. And this physical tension felt like a cornerstone of his personality. In order to release the hold of past judgments and feelings, Enders needed to focus on expansive detachment in his mouth. Through his spiritual practice, he was able to do some emotional and attitudinal healing. Freeing up the tension in his face didn't happen overnight, but it was an essential piece of his spiritual learning.

Annette. Annette drifted in a relaxed state of delicious expansion after each session of bodywork. It felt like she was floating in air, free of all physical encumbrances and at one with all life. She was in a state of Grace. But the moment she became aware of her arms and legs, her critical mind popped the bubble. In both her religious and personal beliefs, the imperfection of her body and divine blessing were at odds. With the coaching of a therapist, Annette was able to let go of her rigid expectations and develop compassion for her body, seeing it truly as an image of God. From this place, she could enjoy spirit space in her body. After all, it was her sensual body that helped her feel the lightness of spirit. Now, being spiritual wasn't just dogma, it was a very up close and personal experience.

Barbara. Barbara was a highly educated, highly cultured woman in her sixties. She'd moved from New York City to the West Coast several years ago and found the nonscientific spiritual perspective of her new friends hard to swallow. As much as she respected her buddies, it seemed like magical thinking to trust the efficacy of anything unseen or unmeasured. This all changed when she started taking yoga classes and followed her instructor's directive to expand her awareness through her body to a limitless sense of connection with all life. As she participated in this ritual week by week, Barbara started to feel a sense of deep inner peace and, yes, connection to something beyond her old beliefs. She didn't need to have scientific proof or a philosophical construct to understand that this was a spiritual experience. It felt as if she'd added a whole new dimension to her life. Looking back, the old way of perceiving reality seemed flat by comparison.

Separating body from spirit has presented a conundrum for seekers throughout time. But what if bringing your body along helped rather than hindered the spiritual journey? What if you didn't have to shed your attachment to the flesh in order to be holy? What if your spiritual direction was about dropping in rather than lifting off? What if living a full life meant being spiritually conscious in your body? The answers to these questions are as straightforward as your flesh and blood. Anytime you breathe and feel the dissolution of boundaries and separateness, your small self becomes part of the greater whole. Any time you tap into your kinesthetic awareness of internal space and external space, your small self becomes part of the greater whole. Any time your body has the sensation of being undifferentiated and continuous with all life, you're no longer attached to the issue of body versus spirit. There is no either/or. All is one. Isn't this just what the spiritual teachers tell us to expect? Isn't this "more space than matter" feeling what quantum physicists are calling reality? Through the subjective experiences of your physical body you can access spirit, soul, atman, *spiritu*, Holy Ghost, or the Great Mystery.

Your spiritual body is a valuable resource and guide for everyday life. It's also a place to find comfort and touch a piece of eternity. Becoming aware of your body's mystical and expansive dimension is like welcoming spirit home. Yet, when you live in a culture that views the body as distinctly material and mechanical, you may need some practice living in sacred space. Pay attention to your spiritual body every day and see if you can feel the presence, hear the voice, touch the wisdom, or experience the ordinary reality of spirit.

Living in sacred space implies that your body *is* sacred. This means it has a quality of transcendence and mystery that can't be deconstructed by science or logic. This means it has a quality of transformation that extends beyond a dense, material experience to an expanded, ethereal experience. Living in sacred space is simply about embracing the "spirit" part of body-mind-spirit. Here are some ways to invite spirit into your life:

Embody Spirit

In this book, you've already learned a couple of good ways to embody spirit in practical ways. Remember how you felt the most mundane moments and most demanding challenges become enlightened when you breathed into them? Just taking a clearing breath at the beginning and end of any activity brings you into the spirit of the moment. Remember how your sense of kinesthetic inner-outer space helped you segue from little self to big self? Just becoming more spacious in any situation invites the presence and power of spirit into anything you do. Just aligning your body with spirit says "I am" and connects you with eternity.

The most profound gift your body can give you is direct access to spirit. Wherever or whenever—driving to work, chatting with friends, shopping, gardening, being intimate, speaking to a large audience, tackling a tough task—you want to infuse a moment or gesture with spirit, all you need to do is breathe, focus, connect, and you've got it! Anytime you feel lost or overwhelmed, remember spirit. Anytime you need to overcome strife, tackle a creative challenge, negotiate a misunderstanding, deal with a crisis or disaster, remember spirit. Anytime you need to show up for an intense personal occasion like birthing, healing, or dying, remember spirit. And, when you're open to it, spirit will come through with the vision, strength, and wisdom you need. Being in your spirit-body makes the difference between feeling scared and feeling sacred.

Honor Spirit

There's a long human history of using ceremony and ritual to honor spirit. Often these include physical gestures such as kneeling, genuflecting, drinking, eating, lighting candles, breaking glasses, etc. Whether the event is traditional or something you've designed yourself, rather than a rote performance, make sure you're actually *in* your body. Being consciously centered in your breathing and connected to inner-outer space means your spirit-body is showing up and participating in the process. In this way, you anchor the importance of the occasion right down to the very core of your being.

Honoring spirit doesn't have to have a reason. Living in sacred space means everything you do is imbued with a focused awareness. You don't have to be restrained by formalities: pause, breathe, connect, and acknowledge the wonder. Show up with honesty and humility. Take a risk, make a friend, create beauty, or be generous. These are all ways to honor spirit. Just taking care of your body, your domicile, or your environment with intention and gratitude is a celebration of spirit. How you approach it makes the difference between the mundane and the sublime. When you honor spirit, does your body feel lighter, easier, bigger, and freer? Perhaps this is the true essence of who you are. Living each day with a sense of spirit creates a sacred context for the journey and a touchstone for body wisdom.

Nine
Body Wisdom for Life

When your smart body shows up, *you* show up. As you've discovered, seeing things from a body-oriented perspective improves every aspect of your life. Rather than cruising on autopilot, you now have an intelligent navigator at the controls. You can rely on your body when it comes to nutrition, exercise, rest, and healing. You can count on your body when it comes to making good decisions and making good impressions. When your smart body weighs in, you know what works for you and what doesn't at the most basic level. Some choices, ideas, opportunities, and relationships resonate and others don't. Your sentient, intuitive body knows the difference.

Yet your smart body showing up is only the beginning—when it happens, your perspective changes and your vision expands. The more you see beyond the narrow horizons of habit and assumption, the more you appreciate your untapped resources. Each time you tap into these resources, you become more body savvy. Living in a smart body is a new way of life. As your experience proves worthy, you will trust your body more and more. Eventually, incorporating your body's point of view becomes a normal way of life.

✿ *Try This: Check In One More Time*

Like most people, until you picked up this book, you probably didn't know the full story about your body. With your head running the show, the notion of trusting, respecting, including, and listening to your body seemed somewhat absurd. Not until your curious mind started to pay attention, experiment, and reconsider, did you know what you were missing. Take a moment to remember why you began reading this book. Did you find what you were seeking? Has your new learning changed your relationship with your body?

- Have your self-care and self-talk become more positive?

- Do you have more ways to handle stress, injury, illness, and discord?

- Do you experience more hope, levity, and peacefulness?

- Is it easier to make decisions and stand in your truth?

- Do you feel more grounded, confident, and effective?

- Is it easier to sense what's going on and feel connected to a
  bigger picture?

Reading this book has given you an opportunity to explore your body's unique intelligence. Step by step, the progressive learning has helped you expand your awareness and embrace the full scope of your potential. As you bore witness to the results over time, the proposition that your body is singularly intelligent and intuitive began to make sense, and even seem logical and natural.

When does your smart body get wise? Perhaps it was a thoughtful friend, pure chance, or an intuitive impulse that put *A Guide to Body Wisdom* in your hands. Something about the title or description appealed to some timely need or interest and you began to read. Perhaps, once you began, a subliminal current reawakened an intelligence that's been there all along. As you delved deeper and experienced your body's unique gifts, you were also developing a body-oriented perspective. You were starting to come to your senses again. As you listened to the sweet and steady presence of your body-voice and followed its guidance, you were also incorporating new information and making it your own. When your smart body offered good counsel, you were listening to a wise ally and mentor. And when your body's sense of space created a bridge to all life, you were aligning your small self with your big self. Looking at the world from a body-oriented perspective is a real paradigm shift.

Your Unique Body of Wisdom

Delightfully, this book doesn't deliver the kind of mixed message where the words tell you one thing and your experience makes you doubt it. Instead, the message is all about paying attention and believing in your body's intelligence. Each concept, each idea, each suggestion is illuminated and validated through the sensibility of your own body. Paying attention establishes your body-mind circuitry. Every time you show up for your body, your body shows up for you. Developing a body-oriented perspective gives you a wider, deeper intuition that seems to come from a deep source of knowing. This is how you grow your unique body of wisdom.

🌸 *Explore: How Has Your Body of Wisdom Grown?*

Reading this book has given you a way to encounter your personal edge. Seeing your everyday reality from a body-oriented perspective probably confirmed some things you already knew. Hopefully, it also nudged you out of your comfort zone and encouraged you to explore new dimensions. The more you participated, the more you learned. As your body-mind was getting smarter, your body wisdom was beginning to percolate.

Take some time to return to your Body Wisdom journal. There's something there for you to see. You don't have to read every word, just skim through to get an idea of where you've been. This is your personal account of how your body wisdom has been growing. After you scan through the journey you've taken, pause for a moment, close your eyes, and tune in one more time (breath/space). Be empty and open and listen for some body wisdom. Ask the following questions:

- What do I know now that I didn't know before?

- Is my idea of my body different?

- Are my self-care routines more effective?

- Do I feel more grounded and focused for relationship and creativity?

- Am I more confident when challenged?

- Has my view of the past, present, and future changed?

Now, put your answers (insights, poems, and drawings) in your journal. Jotting down your insights and discoveries is a good way to assess what you've learned and see how you're making good use of your body wisdom.

✳ *Try This: What's Your Body Wisdom IQ Now?*

Developing a body-oriented perspective has influenced the way you think and live in the world. Chances are you're accessing more of your full potential. Maybe it's time to retake the Body Wisdom IQ Test in chapter 2 and compare the results. Just put your post-test answers right next to the original ones. This is a good way to see the results of the work you've done. And while you're at it, tack on these yes/no questions to see how much body wisdom you've acquired:

- Do you take time to enjoy your physicality and sensual pleasures?

- Do you trust your body to weigh in on day-to-day decisions?

- Can you speak from your body as a source of authority?

- Does your self-talk reflect a high regard for your body?

- Do you bring your heart and spirit along with you to work?

- Do creativity, intimacy, and fun have a high priority?

- Can you find a place of inner peace in the midst of turmoil?

- Does your body feel at one with all life?

This book will have served its purpose if you have a lot of *yes* answers!

Being Body-Wise

Nobody becomes wise without logging a certain amount of qualifying time. You know people who are smart but not particularly wise. Depth, vision, and compassion are cultivated as experience changes your perspective and new behaviors take the place of old. Because wisdom happens over time, it's natural to get wiser as you get older. But listening to your smart body is a way to actively cultivate body wisdom. Any circumstance or situation can be fodder for growth anytime. A challenging health or emotional issue always includes some hidden gems of insight and oversight. The dissolution of a dream or a creative setback can be an opportunity to realign with your inner truth. Hardship can be a way to find compassion and uncover a deeper faith. Ultimately, growing a body of wisdom is your most personal creative act.

No matter when you start, attaining wisdom is a lifelong endeavor. *A Guide to Body Wisdom* has given you all the information and tools you need to keep becoming body-wise. Because you're still alive, there's more growing to do. And your body's here to help you do it.

Mary. As a CPA, Mary knew about keeping accounts in order. But her personal life was a mess. When her health finally broke down, Mary had to address a "self-care deficit." Throughout her life, as she filled the coffers of others, she was emptying her own. Eventually, she became physically, mentally, and spiritually exhausted. Coming to see me was a first step toward changing her priorities and developing self-care skills. Rather than being the problem, Mary's body had taught her a valuable life lesson—you can only give to others what you have already given to yourself. This was a piece of true body wisdom.

Frank. As an athlete, Frank knew his body intimately and counted on it to perform well. Last year, while cross training, he was hit by a car and sustained injuries that took him out of the game. As he tackled a new challenge of healing and repair, his old strategies of working hard and powering through just seemed to make things worse. Not only did his body hurt but his sense of self was suffering as well. Feeling sidelined and scared, he asked me for help. Once he stopped being impatient and demanding, Frank learned to trust his body's healing process and his body began to trust him. And as his healing progressed, he was given a powerful insight. From his body's point of view, it was clear that his impatience was a form of abandonment and his demands were a kind of bullying. When his body recovered and he got back on the field, he decided to bring his "inner coach" along so he could play smart as well as good. This was a piece of true body wisdom.

Elisa. *Elisa moved to New York City for graduate school a week before the 9/11 tragedy. In the months following, she had post-trauma symptoms. Feeling spacey and revved up at the same time, she asked if I could help her focus and relax enough to get back to her studies. It was as if she'd had an out-of-body experience and never came back home. Using the body-centered techniques described in this book, Elisa learned that the sensations of pressure and movement were reassuring reference points no matter where she was or what was happening. Tuning in to the basics of breathing and feeling her body's connection to the earth gave her the comfort and confidence to feel safe again. This was a piece of true body wisdom.*

When have you listened to your body's intuition or inner knowing? Have you ever felt stymied or puzzled and followed your body's feedback to find the opening? Have you ever felt isolated and distressed and embraced your emotional body to find a deeper you? Have you ever had doubts or confusion and trusted your body's essential connection to something bigger and eternal? This is when you really begin to harvest your growing body wisdom.

If you know how to listen in, your body's guidance will outperform any fortune-teller, astrologer, or card reader. If you know how to tune in, your body's intuition will help you circumvent the illusions, distortions, and rationalizations of your mind. If you pay attention, your body will tell you immediately if you are uncomfortable with a situation, uncertain with a decision, or uneasy with a person. Then your rational mind can figure out why this is so. Paying attention to intuition is the key to all good decisions you've made in life; overriding intuition is the source of most bad ones! Likewise, intuition is always an asset when it comes to intimacy. You have the source for true body wisdom at your fingertips and in your heart and gut.

❋ *Explore: True Body Wisdom*

When did you notice your smart body had some wisdom to share? When did you begin to share some of this wisdom with others? I'm sure there's a story or two you could tell. Have you changed your mind about your body? Has your body-oriented perspective simply become part of who you are? If so, this book has done its job. The truth is, your body wisdom has been accumulating since the day you were born and will continue to grow until the day you die. Why not keep this journal going and record it all? When you have an insight or discovery, why not share it with the people you love? Telling others about your discoveries is a good way to own your experience, and they might have some body wisdom to share with you in return.

Hopefully, reading *A Guide to Body Wisdom* has helped you set aside the time and make the effort to discover your smart, wise body. Including this intelligent asset and faithful ally as you go through life will not only mean that you showed up, but that you showed up smart and wise. It won't be long until it just seems natural to live this way all the time. Then, with your embodied confidence, authenticity, and compassion, you can be one of the wisdom keepers.

Troubleshooting Index:
A Guide for Some Common Situations

People seek my professional help for many different reasons. Sometimes they're looking for ways to find more connection and comfort. Sometimes they're seeking a new approach to sleep, anxiety, exhaustion, or motivational problems. Sometimes they want help on a healing journey. And sometimes, their body brings them screaming and crying to my door, seemingly a last resort.

Embracing the wisdom of your body can be the key to resolving dissatisfaction, discomfort, and disease. Once the door is open, you'll have a new perspective and valuable skills to attain your goals. Here's a step-by-step guide to help you customize your exploration to address your specific situation. Just follow the suggested sequence to discover how your wise body can help.

Physical Pain and Chronic Tension

If you need to learn how to negotiate discomfort and maximize comfort, it makes sense to become familiar with the territory.

Begin with

Learn more
Learn to Relax, 88–91
Body Meditation, 93–95
Go Slow, 96

Deepen understanding
Read Healing chapter, 105–135
What Can Tension Tell You? 139

Make a commitment
Everyday Intimacy, 172
Breathing in Spirit Space, 205
Walking Meditation, 208

Sleep Issues

If you need to learn how to get in the sleep zone, your body can help you get there.

Begin with
Checking In, 16–17
Your Breathing Body, 19

Learn more
A Basic Breathing Lesson, 46–48
Rest and Sleep, 63–66
Find Your Sleep Zone, 65

Deepen understanding
Strategies for Letting Go, 82–88
Relax Your Body, 88–90
Relax Your Mind, 90

Make a commitment

Body Breathing, 93
Body Meditation, 93–95
Breathing in Spirit Space, 205

Anxiety

If you need to learn how to get out of your mind, relax, and release, knowing your body is your best strategy.

Begin with

Wake Up, Loosen Up, 15–16
Checking In, 16–17
Your Breathing Body, 19
Communing with Nature, 209–211

Learn more

A Basic Breathing Lesson, 46–48
Five Steps for Emotional Hygiene, 146–148
Get Aligned, 214

Deepen understanding

Rest and Sleep, 63–66
Read Stress and Relaxation chapter, 73–135
Get a Massage, 169

Make a commitment

Spa@Home, 128–129
Breathing in Spirit Space, 206

Mental Overload

If you need to learn how to shift gears and replenish your resources, get out of your head and into your body.

Begin with

Take the Body Wisdom IQ Test, 33–39
Your Personal Health Profile, 44–45
Checking In, 16–17
How's Your Breathing? 46

Learn more

Random Body Checks, 17
A Basic Breathing Lesson, 46–48
Get a Massage, 169

Deepen understanding

Rest and Sleep, 63–66
Read Stress and Relaxation chapter, 73–104

Make a commitment

Spa@Home, 128–129
Breathing in Spirit Space, 205–206
Get in the Spirit, 207–208
Walking Meditation, 208–209

Emotional Upheaval

If you need to find guidance, help, and resolution for emotional times, your feeling body is a trusty companion.

Begin with

Checking In, 16
Follow Your Feelings, 29
A Basic Breathing Lesson, 46–48

Learn more

Deepen understanding

Make a commitment

Injury or Illness

If you need to learn how to make use of your innate resources and return to radiant health, listen to your body.

Begin with

Learn more

Deepen understanding

Make a commitment
Trust Your Body, 42–44
Communing with Nature, 209–211
Injury and Illness, 215–216

Stagnation

If you need to learn how to get it moving again, your moving body can give you the tools and show you the way.

Begin with
Wake Up, Loosen Up, 15–16
Conscious Body, 17–19
Moving, 51–54

Learn more
A Basic Breathing Lesson, 46–48
Emotion is Moving Energy, 144–145
Fork in the Road, 191–192

Deepen understanding
Take the Body Wisdom IQ Test, 33–39
Read the Intimacy and Intuition chapter, 163–201

Make a commitment
Aesthetics, 67–71
Focused Moving/Take Your Body for a Walk, 95–96
Breathing in Spirit Space, 205
Get in the Spirit, 207–208

Uncertainty Regarding Future

If you need to listen to your inner-knowing and trust the unknown, knowing your body will help you proceed with confidence.

Begin with

Learn more

Deepen understanding

Make a commitment

Low Energy or Boredom

If you need to reboot and recharge, listen to your body to renew your enthusiasm and rekindle your interest.

Begin with

Learn more

Breathing, 46–48

Lighten Up, 99

Deepen understanding

Take the Body Wisdom IQ Test, 33–39

Fitness, 54–57

Enjoy Life, 87–88

Make a commitment

Wake Up, Loosen Up, 15–16

Walking Meditation, 208–209

Spa@Home, 128–129

Negative Self-Talk, Low Self-Esteem

If you need to align with your highest potential and manifest the positive, pay attention and listen to your aware body.

Begin with

How Do You Stand? 24–25

Body-Home Tour, 13–14

Changing Your Mind/Listen In, 27–29

Learn more

Rest and Sleep, 63–66

Enjoy Life, 87–88

Emotional Posture, 139–140

Five Steps for Emotional Hygiene, 146–148

Deepen understanding

Read Waking Up chapter, 9–32

Give Yourself a Little Love, 167–168

Your Conscious Body, 17–19

Make a commitment
Being Present, 14–15
Get a Massage, 169–170
Living in Sacred Space, 218–220

Old Habits and Addictions

Recovering from old habits and addictions is a form of physical-emotional-spiritual healing. Developing body-oriented perspective will help you stay the course and find success.

Begin with
Start at the Beginning, 10–19
What's Your Assignment?, 107–108
River of Life, 120–122

Learn more
Read Healing chapter, 105–135
What Can Tension Tell You? 139
Emotional Posture, 139–140
What's Your Posture Holding? 140–141
Your Healing Journey, 122–123

Deepen understanding
History Leaves an Impression, 21–23
Go Slow, 96–97
Find the Gift, 115–116
Understanding the Emotional Body, 144
Read Body and Spirit chapter, 203–221

Make a commitment
Changing Your Mind/Listening In, 27–29
An Attitude of Gratitude, 132
Create Ceremony, 132–135

Self-Confidence

If you want to put your best foot forward and stand in your power, your body's here to help you.

Begin with

Your Conscious Body, 17–19

How Do You Stand? 24–25

Body-Talk, 176

Learn more

Your Stress Footprint, 81–82

A Basic Breathing Lesson, 46–47

Become Aware, 82–83

Finding Neutral, 152

Read The Emotional Body chapter, 137–162

Deepen understanding

Tune In to Personal Space, 173

How Do You Face the World? 101

Intuition for Social Success, 197–198

Intuition for Business, 198–199

Make a commitment

Tips for Good Communication, 177

Get Aligned, 214–215

Being Body-Wise, 227–228

Give and Receive Love

Tuning in to your sensible body makes all the difference if you want to show up for love 100 percent.

Begin with

Learn more

Deepen understanding

Make a commitment

Inspiration

If you're looking for a reliable portal to inspiration and insight, let your body show you the way.

Begin with

Learn more

Deepen understanding

Make a commitment

Perspective

If you need to broaden your vision and see the forest as well as the tress, get out of your mind and trust your body-sense.

Begin with

Learn more

Deepen understanding

Change Your Mindset, 83–84

An Attitude of Gratitude, 132

Emotion Is Moving Energy, 144–145

Intuition Practicum, 190–201

Make a commitment

Enjoy Life, 87–88

Lighten Up, 99

Feel the Wonder, 206

Existential Crisis

Your ageless, timeless body can anchor you in present time when you feel adrift and uncertain. It also connects you to your deepest wisdom and instinctual knowing.

Begin with

Consider Your Balance, 45

Rest and Sleep, 63–66

Change Your Mindset, 83–84

Learn more

Emotion Is Moving Energy, 145–146

A Basic Breathing Lesson, 46–48

Intuition for Changing Times, 200

Deepen understanding

Do You Have Body Sense? 26–27

Your Stress Footprint, 81–82

Relaxation, 88–92

Read Body and Spirit chapter, 203–221

Make a commitment
Checking In, 16–17
Communing with Nature, 209–211
Ask for a Hug, 168–169

Spiritual Connection

When you tune in, your body can be a gateway to spiritual awareness.

Begin with
Give Your Mind Something to Do, 12
Open Your Mind, 204
Get Aligned, 214–215

Learn more
What Is Body Wisdom? 31–32
Spirit Lives in the Body Too, 30–31
Intuition for the Spiritual Journey, 200–201

Deepen understanding
Take Your Body for a Walk, 95–96
Tune In to Personal Space, 173
Sharing Silence, 178–179
Read Body and Spirit chapter, 203–221

Make a commitment
Limit Exposure, 86–87
Body Meditation, 93–95
Breathing in Spirit Space, 205–206
Feel the Wonder, 206
Living in Sacred Space, 218–220

Once your immediate needs have been addressed, it'll be easier to focus on becoming body-wise in every aspect of life. *A Guide to Body Wisdom* is full of practical information and exercises to help you find comfort, fulfillment, and delight in your wise body.

Bibliography

Journal Articles

Chittaranjan, Andrade. "Prayer and Healing: A Medical and Scientific Perspective on Randomized Controlled Trials," *Indian Journal of Psychiatry,* Oct–Dec 2009. www.ncbi.nlm.nih.gov/pmc/articles/PMC2802370.

Hunt, Valerie V. "Study of Structural Integration from Neuromuscular, Energy Field, and Emotional Approaches," accessed Aug 2017. www.somatics.de, www.somatics.de/artikel/for-professionals/2-article/96-study-of -structural-integrations.from.neuromuscular-energy-field-and -emotional-approaches.

Woodyard, Catherine. "Exploring the Therapeutic Effects of Yoga and Its Ability to Increase Quality of Life." *International Journal of Yoga,* Jul–Dec 2011. ncbi.nlm.nih.gov/pmc/articles/PMC193654/.

News or Magazine Articles

Ambrosia, Gloria Taraniya. "The Experience of Feeling." Barre Center for Buddhist Studies Spring newsletter, 2000. www.bcbsdharma.org/article /the-experience-of-feeling-insight-into-the-aggregates/.

Brodwin, Erin, Jessica Orwig, and Dina Spector. "How to Feel Happier, According to Neuroscientists and Psychologists." *Business Insider,* July 11, 2017. uk.businessinsider.com/how-fee-happy-happier-better-2017-7.html.

Brown, Kristin V. "How Posture Influences Mood, Energy, and Thoughts." *SF Gate*, September 3, 2013. sfgate.com/health/article/How-posture -influences-mood-energy-thoughts-4784543.php.

Chatterjee, Anjan. "The Aesthetic Brain." *Oxford Scholarship Online*, January 2014. www.oxfordscholarship.com/view/10.1093/acprof:oso /9780199811809.001.0001/acprof-9780199811809.

Cook, Gareth. "The Science of Healing Thoughts." *Scientific American*, January 19, 2016. www.scientificamerican.com/article/the-science-of-healing -thoughts/.

De Lang, Catherine. "The Unsung Sense: How Smell Rules Your Life." *New Science,* September 2011. www.newscientist.com/article/mg21128301 -800-the-unsung-sense-how-smell-rules-your-life/.

Gholipour, Bahar. "Happily Surprised! People Use More Facial Expressions Than Thought." *Live Science-Health*, March 31, 2014. www.livescience.com /44494-human-facial-expressions-compound-emotions.html.

Howes, Ryan. "Laughter in Therapy." *Psychology Today*, December 31, 2013. www.psychologytoday.com/blog/in-therapy/201312/laughter-in-therapy .html.

Lapowsky, Issie. "Don't Multitask: Your Brain Will Thank You." *Time,* April 17, 2013. www.business.time.com/2013/04/17/dont-multitask-your-brain-will -thank-you/.

Lehrer, Jonah. "The Eureka Hunt." *New Yorker,* July 28, 2008. www.newyorker .com/magazine/2008/07/28/the-eureka-hunt.htms.

Liebertz, Charmaine. "Want Clear Thinking? Relax." *Scientific American Mind,* October 1, 2005. www.scientificamerican.com/article/want-clear -thinking-relax.html.

Ohikuare, Judith. "How Actors Create Emotions: A Problematic Psychology." *Atlantic,* March 10, 2014. www.theatlantic.com/health/archive/2014/03/ how-actors-createmotions-a problematic-psychology/284291/.

Root-Bernstein, Michele, and Robert Root-Bernstein. "Einstein on Creative Thinking." *Psychology Today*, March 31, 2010. www.psychologytoday.com /blog/imagine/201003/einstein-creative-thinking-music-and-the -intuitive-art-scientific-imagination.

Sonnenburg, Justin, and Erica Sonnenburg. "Gut Feelings—the 'Second Brain' in Our Gastrointestinal Systems [Excerpt]" *Scientific American,* May 2015. www.scientificamerican.com/article/gut-feelings-the-second-brain-in-our -gastrointestinal-systems-excerpt/.

Walia, Arjun. "How Your Aura Affects Your Health and Those Around You." *Collective Evolution,* February 10, 2016. www.collective-evolution .com/2016/02/10/this-is-how-your-aura-affects-your-health-those-around -you.htms.

Wellcome Trust. "Everybody Laughs, Everybody Cries: Researchers Identify Universal Emotions." *Science Daily,* January 26, 2010. www.sciencedaily .com/releases/2010/01/100125173234.htm.

Whitbourne, Susan Krause. "What Your Most Vivid Memories Say About You." *Psychology Today*, November 20, 2012. www.psychologytoday.com /blog/fulfillment-any-age/201211/what-your-most-vivid-memories-say -about-you.html.

Williams, Ray. "Slowing Down Can Increase Productivity and Happiness." *Psychology Today*, June 17, 2014. www.psychologytoday.com/blog/wired -success/201406/slowing-down-can-increase-productivity-and-happiness -part-1.html.

Website Content

BrainyQuote.com, s.v. "Pierre Teilhard de Chardin." Accessed August 15, 2017. www.brainyquote.com/quotes.p.pierreteil160888.

Cuddy, Amy. "Your Body Language May Shape Who You Are." Video filmed June 2012 at TEDGlobal, 20:19. www.ted.com/amy_cuddy_your_body _language_shapes_who_your_are?share=1c7ca032el.

Help Guide. "Stress Symptoms, Signs, and Causes." Accessed May, 2016. www.helpguide.org/articles/stress/stress-symptoms-signs-and-causes.htm.

Mayo Clinic staff. "Stress Symptoms: Effects on Your Body and Behavior." Accessed May 2017, www.mayoclinic.org/healthy-lifestyle/stress -management/in-depth/stress-symptoms/art-20050987.html.

NIH News in Health. "Hugs and Cuddles Have Long-Term Effects." Last modified February 2007. newsinhealth.nih.gov/2007/february/docs/01features _01.html.

Spiritual Competency Resource Center. "Spiritual Emergence," Lesson 3.1. Accessed April 2017. www.spiritualcompentency.com/dsm4/lesson3 _1.asp.

Resource Guide

Website
Learn more about Ann Todhunter Brode and Body Wisdom for Life.
....
www.anntodhunterbrode.com

Facebook
Keep up to date on Ann's calendar of events and tidbits of pertinent body wisdom.
....
www.facebook.com/bodywisdomforlife

Body Wisdom Blog and Mini-Posts
Subscribe to these short, inspiring email pieces and informative blog posts featuring a body-mind topic, insights and science, and practical ways to be body-wise.
....
www.anntodhunterbrode.com/follow

Audio
Body Breath: Three Guided Meditations to help you relax and focus.
....
www.anntodhunterbrode.com/media

Instructional Videos

Brode has designed several instructional videos to facilitate some of the concepts in this book. Wake Up, Loosen Up, S.L.E.E.P. , and more.

....

www.anntodhunterbrode.com/media

Aston Kinetics

Judith Aston has produced several videos to explain simple movement principles and the ergonomics of walking, sitting, support, alignment, and more.

....

www.astonkinetics.com/instructional-videos

Share Your Stories

I'm interested in your body wisdom journey. Just like the anecdotal stories in this book, your discoveries and insights could be very helpful to others. Here's how we can share them:

- Jot down what you've learned, share your stories, personal insights, and healing epiphanies

- Include your permission to publish the account

- Copy, paste, and format as an email

- Send to ann@annbrode.com

GET MORE AT LLEWELLYN.COM

Visit us online to browse hundreds of our books and decks, plus sign up to receive our e-newsletters and exclusive online offers.

- Free tarot readings • Spell-a-Day • Moon phases
- Recipes, spells, and tips • Blogs • Encyclopedia
- Author interviews, articles, and upcoming events

GET SOCIAL WITH LLEWELLYN

Find us on **f**   **y** @LlewellynBooks

www.Facebook.com/LlewellynBooks

GET BOOKS AT LLEWELLYN

LLEWELLYN ORDERING INFORMATION

 Order online: Visit our website at www.llewellyn.com to select your books and place an order on our secure server.

 Order by phone:
- Call toll free within the US at 1-877-NEW-WRLD (1-877-639-9753)
- We accept VISA, MasterCard, American Express, and Discover.
- Canadian customers must use credit cards.

✉ **Order by mail:**
Send the full price of your order (MN residents add 6.875% sales tax) in US funds plus postage and handling to: Llewellyn Worldwide, 2143 Wooddale Drive, Woodbury, MN 55125-2989

POSTAGE AND HANDLING

STANDARD (US):
(Please allow 12 business days)
$30.00 and under, add $6.00.
$30.01 and over, FREE SHIPPING.

INTERNATIONAL ORDERS,
INCLUDING CANADA:
$16.00 for one book, plus $3.00 for each additional book.

Visit us online for more shipping options. Prices subject to change.

FREE CATALOG!

To order, call
1-877-
NEW-WRLD
ext. 8236
or visit our
website

new worlds
Reaping
Personal Power
Every Day

GHASTLY
LIVING AS A
MAGICKAL FAMILY
AND MORE!

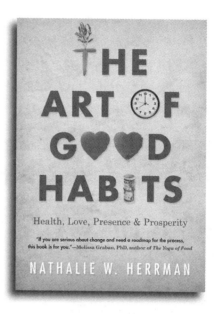

THE ART OF G♥♥D HAB♦TS

Health, Love, Presence & Prosperity

"If you are serious about change and need a roadmap for the process,
this book is for you."—Melissa Grabau, PhD, author of *The Yoga of Food*

NATHALIE W. HERRMAN

The Art of Good Habits
Health, Love, Presence & Prosperity
Nathalie W. Herrman

Take ownership of your happiness through simple but effective changes to the way you approach health, love, presence, and prosperity. *The Art of Good Habits* presents a step-by-step action plan to achieve your goals and maintain them for continued success.

Join Nathalie W. Herrman on a life-changing journey toward wellness and satisfaction using this remarkable book as your road map. Gain empowerment and control over life's challenges with effective exercises and easy-to-understand principles. Discover how to look within yourself for answers and change your habits for the better. With this book's four-pillar system—honesty, willingness, awareness, and appreciation—you'll unlock the power of enlightened living.

978-0-7387-4600-5, 5 x 7, 264 pp.   **$16.99**

To order, call 1-877-NEW-WRLD
Prices subject to change without notice
Order at Llewellyn.com 24 hours a day, 7 days a week!

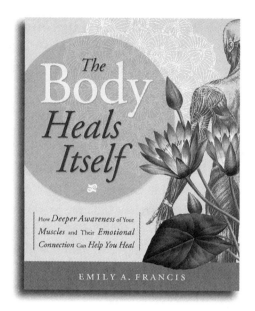

The Body Heals Itself

How *Deeper Awareness* of Your *Muscles* and Their *Emotional Connection* Can *Help You Heal*

EMILY A. FRANCIS

The Body Heals Itself
How Deeper Awareness of Your Muscles and Their Emotional Connection Can Help You Heal
Emily A. Francis

You know a lot about the emotions in your mind and heart, but you probably don't know much about the emotions in your muscle body. The muscles are storehouses of emotion, and pain in those muscles is how your body reveals what needs to be healed—both emotionally and physically. Organized by muscle groups, *The Body Heals Itself* is your ideal guide to understanding the link between your emotions and muscle bodies.

This book acts as a road map for the energetic journey within your own body, showing you how to recognize and release stored emotions to let go of pain. You'll discover which emotions are often paired with a specific muscle area and how muscles speak of everything from past traumas to current celebrations. Using stretches, affirmations, visualizations, and more, Emily A. Francis teaches you to unite your mind and body for better health and emotional well-being.

978-0-7387-5073-6, 7½ x 9¼, 312 pp.   **$21.99**

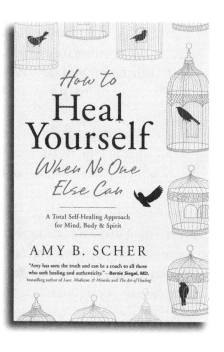

How to
Heal
Yourself
When No One
Else Can

A Total Self-Healing Approach
for Mind, Body & Spirit

AMY B. SCHER

"Amy has seen the truth and can be a coach to all those
who seek healing and authenticity."—**Bernie Siegel, MD,**
bestselling author of *Love, Medicine, & Miracles* and *The Art of Healing*

How to Heal Yourself When No One Else Can
A Total Self-Healing Approach for Mind, Body & Spirit
Amy B. Scher

Using energy therapy and emotional healing techniques, *How to Heal Yourself When No One Else Can* shows you how to achieve complete and permanent healing by loving, accepting, and being yourself no matter what. Energy therapist Amy Scher presents an easy-to-understand, three-part approach to removing blockages, changing your relationship with stress, and coming into alignment with who you truly are.

After overcoming a life-threatening illness, Amy had an epiphany that healing is more than just physical. Her dramatic story serves as a powerful example of how beneficial it is to address our emotional energies, particularly when nothing else works. Discover areas of imbalance and easy ways to address them on your healing journey. Whether you are experiencing physical symptoms or are just feeling lost, sad, anxious, or emotionally unbalanced, this book can change your life.

978-0-7387-4554-1, 6 x 9, 288 pp.   **$17.99**

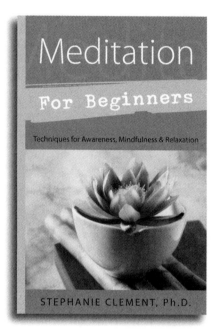

Meditation

For Beginners

Techniques for Awareness, Mindfulness & Relaxation

STEPHANIE CLEMENT, Ph.D.

Meditation for Beginners
Techniques for Awareness, Mindfulness & Relaxation
Stephanie Clement, PhD

Break the barrier between your conscious and unconscious minds.

Perhaps the greatest boundary we set for ourselves is the one between the conscious and less conscious parts of our own minds. We all need a way to gain deeper understanding of what goes on inside our minds when we are awake, asleep, or just not paying attention. Meditation is one way to pay attention long enough to find out.

Meditation for Beginners offers a step-by-step approach to meditation, with exercises that introduce you to the rich possibilities of this age-old spiritual practice. Improve concentration, relax your body quickly and easily, work with your natural healing ability, and enhance performance in sports and other activities. Just a few minutes each day is all that's needed.

978-0-7387-0203-2, 5³⁄₁₆ x 8, 264 pp.   **$14.99**

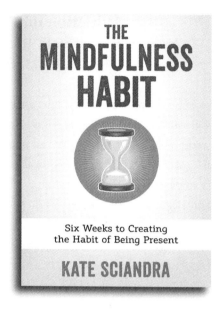

THE MINDFULNESS HABIT

Six Weeks to Creating
the Habit of Being Present

KATE SCIANDRA

The Mindfulness Habit
Six Weeks to Creating the Habit of Being Present
KATE SCIANDRA

This step-by-step book offers a demystified and non-time-consuming approach to being present. It addresses the difference between meditation and mindfulness, why mindfulness is important, and dispels common misconceptions about the process. It then takes a step-by-step approach to not only teach exercises and techniques for developing mindfulness, but also includes instructions for finding the everyday opportunities to put them in place. This is done in a way that uses habit-forming principles so that at the end of six weeks, you have both a tool kit and a habit for using it regularly.

The Mindfulness Habit helps you understand the value of living in the moment and offers many ways to create the habit of finding opportunities for mindfulness. In each section of the book, you'll discover information about a variety of topics, exercises and instructions for building mindful habits in your life, and much more.

978-0-7387-4189-5, 5 x 7, 216 pp. $16.99
